MW01278626

So, Where's My Girlfriend?

So, Where's My Girlfriend?

www.sowheresmygirlfriend.com

by Mark Rainier

Hey Tina,
Save this book ... it
might be worth
something one day!

- Mark

First Edition
ISBN: 978-0-9813361-0-7

So, Where's My Girlfriend?

Thanks to

Gloria, Linda, Lisa, Josephine, Alissa, Howard and Tat for always helping me out.

So, Where's My Girlfriend?

Table of Contents

So, Where's My Girlfriend?

Introduction

Hi.

I have a friend named James whom I met a long time ago.

James was a man who was very accomplished in his career and education. He went to a posh private school and proceeded to a well-known university. Upon graduating, James got a good job that paid a handsome salary. Today, James lives in a beautiful, upscale condominium in the heart of the city. His hobbies include photography and cooking. I hear he makes a great butternut squash soup.

It seems that James is a happy camper in life since he lives a life many people would envy. Hell, I envy his life. You should see the size of his television.

If life has been so good to James, why wouldn't he be happy?

Well, the truth of the matter is: James is deathly miserable.

James is miserable because he can't get any girls.

He doesn't have a girlfriend and has never had sex, making him one frustrated virgin.

How do I know all of this?

Well, he's infatuated with this girl named Christine.

Christine told me. This is what she said:

Her: *"You know, James is a really nice guy."*

Me: *"Really?"*

Her: *"Yes. He's so nice and caring. I don't get why he can't get any girls?"*

Me: *"He sounds like a good guy to me. I don't see how he can't get any girls."*

Her: *"Well, he can't. He's 29 and he's still a virgin."*

Me: *"How do you know that he's still a virgin?"*

Her: *"He told me."*

Me: *"Maybe it's a values issue, like he's saving himself for his wedding night".*

Her: *"Oh no. He wants to lose it badly. I feel so bad for him. He's such a nice guy!"*

Me: *"Then why don't you go out with him?"*

Her: *"Oh, no…he's just not for me"*

What a tragedy.

Oh yeah, Christine told me all of this as we were lying in bed.

So, Where's My Girlfriend?

By the way, I'm not as well-off as James. (Hell, I drive a Corolla) and I certainly can't make butternut squash soup as good as James. On paper, James is clearly more attractive than me but in reality, this guy's striking out while I'm hitting for the cycle.

So, what happened?

This is the sad truth about this world: a man can be a great success in every other sphere of his life but if he's a failure in his personal relationships, then his entire life is considered a failure. You see, society discriminates against single people. In restaurants, seats for single people are usually located at the bar so that they don't spoil the appetite of couples and families. If they do have seating for single people, it's usually located by the restroom. In Disneyland, some rides actually have two lines: one line is the regular line and the other line is for "single seat riders". The "single seat rider" line is for people who show up to Disneyland by themselves and have no one to sit with for the roller coaster rides. These poor souls get to ride only when there's an odd empty seat. You can say that these people are the odds and ends of the equation. In other words, single people are the hot dogs of this world. Sure, it's fine to be single when you're young but when you see yourself slowly going up the hill of Life, it's only downhill afterwards.
As well, being single is a time-sensitive status: if a girl is young and single, then she's "playing the field". If she's old and single, then she's a cougar. For guys, a young bachelor is "a player" while an older, single man is "the creepy uncle that shows up during Thanksgiving."
The reason is that the relationship between guys and girls is not an exact science and figuring out the opposite sex is probably harder than rocket science. This is why chick flicks still exist, Sarah Jessica Parker still has work and you're holding this book: Everyone always thinks that they need help in the relationship department especially if they're single. No one is born knowing how to date or how to hold steady relationships. Being successful with the opposite sex is so important; they should teach gender relations in school right before calculus and after history.
In the case of poor James, it's not completely his fault that he couldn't get Christine. What James never realized is that girls are never direct. They are always subtle. I believe

that girls are always too polite to give a guy the brutal truth. Notice how Christine heavily promoted James' good qualities but when faced with the prospect of actually going out with him, she politely balked. She was saying that a girl should go out with James, just not her. I believe that this type of confusion contributes to an awful amount of miscommunication between guys and girls. This is what happens: Christine treats James strictly as a friend. So being a good friend, Christine tries to keep James' spirits up by constantly praising and complimenting him. James however thinks he's reading between the lines and believes that she's into him. Girls can live with the idea of maintaining a non-sexual/non romantic relationship with guys. Most girls can eliminate the idea of a romantic relationship with a guy permanently in their head. Usually one event, character flaw or situation may occur that disqualifies the guy from being boyfriend material forever. For example, he gets caught masturbating to her Facebook pictures and suddenly he's an "asshole" or a "pervert". What kind of injustice is that?

Guys on the other hand, only temporary suspend potential romance in their head until the situation changes. For guys, the possibility of going out with a girl is always in the back of their heads. For example, Bob dates Sally. Bob is then introduced to Sally's best friend, Judy. As long as Bob is dating Sally, he will temporary suspend romantic possibilities for Judy. If the situation changes however (i.e. break up with Sally), Bob will then go after Judy with romantic intentions. On the other hand, Judy will find Bob to be creepy because Judy had permanently disqualified him as boyfriend material the first time she was introduced to him by Sally.

Guys never understand this girl logic and will only think that Judy is just playing hard to get. After a few futile attempts to get into Judy's pants however Bob will probably move on. This is because guys are lazy (I'll talk about lazy guys later in the book).

Finally, despite what moral values parents and religious organizations try to instill in people, the ugly truth still prevails: looks matter heavily in this world. So, I forgot to mention another thing about James: he's not a very attractive guy. As much as people would like to say that looks are not important to them, nobody wants to marry an ugly person. I have never heard a woman say: "*I hope I marry an ugly man so I can have ugly babies.*" It can be clearly seen that society values attractive people. Studies have proven that attractive people tend to make more money than less attractive (ugly) people. At the

So, Where's My Girlfriend?

same time, attractive people are more liked by other people therefore it is probably in everybody's best interest to be attractive.

To sum up, there are three things I hope you just learned: Firstly, being single is heavily affected by time. Secondly, girls are subtle creatures and operate completely opposite from guys. Thirdly, there are some things in this world that are crucial in attracting the opposite sex (looks is one of them). Remember these themes as they will keep popping up throughout this book.

Now, I want you to think about Leon Lett.

Leon Lett was an American football player who played eleven seasons for the Dallas Cowboys. He played Defensive Tackle and he was quite good at what he did. During his time in the NFL, he was a three-time Super Bowl Champion and was selected to the Pro Bowl twice. Despite all the good plays he made throughout his career, Leon Lett will always be remembered for two boneheaded plays he made in his career during two nationally televised games.

The first bonehead play he made was to show off during the Super Bowl. As explained on Wikipedia:

"Late in the fourth quarter, Lett made a play by recovering a fumble on Buffalo's 45 yard line and proceeded to run it back towards the endzone. When he reached the 10- yard line, he started to slow, and held the ball out as he approached the goal line. However, he didn't see a hustling Don Beebe, who was chasing him down from behind. Beebe knocked the ball out of Lett's outstretched hand just before he crossed the goal line, which sent the ball through the endzone, and resulted in a touchback that cost Lett his touchdown. Lett later said he was watching the Jumbotron, and trying to do a "Michael Irvin", where he put the ball out across the goal line.

The Cowboys had a commanding 52-17 lead at the time, and the play did not affect the outcome of the game, but it certainly embarrassed Lett, and it is still well known by football fans today. Lett's gaffe also cost the Cowboys the record for most points scored

So, Where's My Girlfriend?

*in a Super Bowl (55, by the San Francisco 49ers in Super Bowl XXIV), and may have
cost Dallas the largest margin of victory in a Super Bowl."*

Truly, Leon did a remarkably regrettable thing. If you don't understand football, Mr. Lett
pretty much did something stupid.

This was the second bonehead play committed by Leon:

*The second play (ranked #3 in both ESPN lists) occurred during the very next season and
was actually more serious as it resulted in a Cowboy defeat. On Thanksgiving Day in
1993, during a rare snow and sleet storm in Dallas, the Cowboys were leading the Miami
Dolphins 14-13 with mere seconds remaining in the game. The Dolphins attempted a 41-
yard field goal to take the lead but the kick was blocked. While most of his teammates
began celebrating, Lett attempted to recover the ball but slipped on the ice as he
attempted to pick the football up, and Miami recovered the "muff" on the Dallas one yard
line. There was no need to pick up the ball as the Cowboys would have automatically
received possession and could have simply run out the clock. By touching the ball and
then failing to hold onto it, Lett enabled the Dolphins to take possession and then try
another field goal. This second attempt was successful and the Dolphins won the game
16-14.*

In fact, among ESPN's *25 Biggest Sports Blunders* two of the top three blunders are
attributed to Lett. The fans ranked him #1 and #3 biggest failure of all time. With
rankings like that, it's no wonder that Leon's Super Bowl Championship rings and his
ProBowl selections never come up in people's heads when his name comes up. His name
will forever be associated with those two failures.

The football career of Leon Lett is a clear example of how a series of unfortunate events
can wipe out a lifetime of success.

In terms of dating, I believe that a few bad incidences involving a girl can permanently
ruin a guy's self-image and self esteem which will probably lead to a lifetime of crippling
impotence and a dedicated subscription to pornfidelity.com. In this society, a gentleman's

So, Where's My Girlfriend?

manhood is often judged by how many girls he can attract. Sure, he can make six figures but that won't amount to jackshit if he can't get a girl (well, not completely true if he can afford an escort but we'll save that discussion for another time).

As my man Al Pacino says in the movie *Scarface*:

"In this country, you gotta make the money first. Then when you get the money, you get the power. Then when you get the power, then you get the women"

There's pretty much no point in getting the money and the power if you can't get the women to help boost your gigantic ego for being rich and your anemic level of self-respect for being a rich, corporate sell-out. To repeat, society has made it unacceptable for men to be considered successful in life unless they have an impressive record of dating to match their impressive bank account. For those that are naturally suave, this isn't a problem. For the majority of us who aren't naturals however, this is a major problem.

So what can the unsuave do?
 What else?

They learn.

The things I have just discussed are just the tip of the iceberg on the knowledge I have acquired throughout my years of dating and talking to girls. I wrote this book for three reasons: the first one is to amuse myself while the second reason is to entertain other people. Finally the third reason for writing this book is to help people find their loved ones, so that no one will ever have to eat by the bar or sit by themselves on a roller coaster at Disneyland.

So, Where's My Girlfriend?

How Many Fish are Really in the Sea?

I think we're all familiar with the saying *"There's plenty of fish in the sea"*
I hope you realize that this saying has nothing to do with fishermen (although it
technically can, since women always love seamen). Instead, this is what my buddies tell
me when a girl rejects me:

Me: *So she finally signed that restraining order*
Buddy: *Ah...there's plenty of fish in the sea*

Me: *So she finally tattooed* **"I don't love YOU anymore, Mark"** *on her forehead*
Buddy: *Ah...there's plenty of fish in the sea*

I actually read somewhere that if the world's population is at 6.8 billion, and we assume
that 50% of the population are females, then there's about 3.4 billion girls out there for
me. So the rationale is as follows:
"There's plenty of fish in the sea, specifically 3.4 billion girls for me"
I started thinking about this. One night, I said:
"Are there really 3.4 billion girls for me?"
I wanted to know so I decided to find out using some deductive thinking.

1. If there are 6.8 billion people in the world, we will assume 50% are female
= **3.4 billion girls for me**

2. Within this 3.4 billion, we'll assume that 25% are under the age of 18 therefore I am
not legally allowed near them (underaged = Prison term) (19+ = let's take you to
McDonald's!)
= 3.4 billion x 25% = 850,000,000
= 3.4 billion - 850,000,000
= **2 550 000 000 girls for me**

So, Where's My Girlfriend?

3. Within the 2.55 billion, we'll assume that 55% are 40+ years old (arbitrary age - if the girl is still hot at 40, then why not?) I chose 55% since statistics show that people are living longer and we have this upside pyramid in terms of age patterns so I'm assuming that more than half of people are 40+ years old.

= 2.55 billion x 55% = 1 402 500 000

= 2.55 billion - 1 402 500 000

= **1 147 500 000 girls for me**

4. Within the 1.147 billion plus, we'll say that 40% of the girls are married and intend to stay married (it just takes too much effort to sneak around behind the husband's back – I'm sick of hiding under the bed):

= 1 147 500 000 x 40% = 459 000 000

= 1 147 500 000 - 405 000 000

= **688 500 000 girls for me**

5. Within the 688 500 000, we'll assume that 40% are co-habitating/engaged to their soul mates and have no intention of leaving.

= 688 500 000 x 40%

= 688 500 000 – 275 400 000

= **413 100 000 girls for me**

6. Within the 413 100 000, we'll assume that 15% of girls are only interested in girls

= 413 100 000 x 15%

= 413 100 000 – 61 965 000

= **351 135 000 girls for me**

7. Within the 351 135 000, we'll say that 5% are into hard drugs and Satan Worship (Yeah, I know that I shouldn't judge but I don't want to wake up one day tied up and sacrificed to the Dark Prince)

= 351 135 000 x 5%

= 351 135 000 - 17 556 750

So, Where's My Girlfriend?

= 333 578 250 girls for me

8. Within the 333 578 250, we'll say that 15% are obsessed with marrying someone…anyone…as long as the guy breathes and can wiggle his fingers.
= 333 578 250 x 15%
= 333 578 250 - 50 036 737
= 283 541 513 girls for me

9. Within the 283 541 513, we'll say that another 15% of girls don't know what they want in a relationship thereby pissing me off
= 283 541 513 x 15%
= 283 541 513 – 42 531 227
= 241 010 286 girls for me

10. Within the 241 010 286, we'll say that 5% have caught me staring at them on the subway/mall thereby eliminating any chances I have of ever going out with them:
=241 010 286 x 5%
=241 010 286 – 12 050 514
= 228 959 772 girls for me

11. Within the 228 959 772, 40% of these girls fought immaturity…and immaturity won.
= 228 959 772 x 40%
= 228 959 772 – 96 404 114
= 144 606 172 girls for me

12. Within the 144 606 172, we'll say a good 90% of girls like to play hard-to-get and expect me to chase them only to find out that she's the only one playing this silly game of hide and seek. I told you guys are lazy.
= 144 606 172 x 90%
= 144 606 172 – 130 145 555
= 14 460 617 girls for me

So, Where's My Girlfriend?

There you have it. After a rigorous, scientific analysis (that included jotting down numbers on the back of a napkin), it appears that when people say *'Plenty of Fish'*, they really mean about 14 million girls. So, if I plan to get married by let's say...35, then I have about 9 years to meet 14 million girls. So, I have to try and meet 1.5 million girls per year.

If I can give up sleeping and meaningful employment, then this might be possible. At the same time, I can learn sign language so that I can literally talk to multiple girls at the same time. I can verbally say one thing to one, while I furiously sign to another.

The bottom line is clear: there's a lot of fish in the ocean.

The following stories are about 12 of those fish.

So, Where's My Girlfriend?

The Stories

Note: All names used in these stories are fake so that I won't get kicked in the nuts.

So, Where's My Girlfriend?

My First Kiss of Death

I think that the best way to tell you all about my experiences with the female gender is to probably start right from the beginning and tell you about the first time I kissed someone other than my grandmother. This is a story about my first "girlfriend" whom I met during high school. I generously use quotation marks to describe her as my girlfriend because she didn't really act like one. In fact, we only "went out" for one whole month before she ended things. To add insult to injury, during that entire time we were officially dating, I hardly ever saw her. All we did was talk on the phone therefore I never got the chance to see her, hug her or sex her. Thank God I was already heavily into porn at that time so that kept me busy for a while. Even though I didn't get to hug her or sleep with her, let me tell you about that time I tried to kiss her…

Amanda was a girl I met during high school. She was quite the petite girl at about 5'3 and weighing about 90 lbs. She had black shoulder-length straight hair (which was tied in a pony tail when she felt adventurous) and wore glasses and pants all the time. She was the type of girl that didn't believe in make-up and looked the same whether she was in physics class or at a club. Let's just say that if she were an ice cream flavor, she'd be vanilla. At that time, I was ecstatic since there was a girl who actually liked me. I guess there's a first time for everything and I was about to get my first taste of a relationship albeit a dysfunctional one.

Experiencing a relationship for the very first time is very risky, since there are no other previous relationships to compare it to. When you don't have a previous relationship to compare something to, you might think that anything that happens is okay and whatever transpires during that relationship is supposed to be normal. I guess that thinking sort of works, like when parents mercilessly beat their children and tell them it's for their own good. I felt that I endured a lot of mental abuse during the time I was with Amanda. Specifically she would say things that would drive me ape shit, like talk lovingly about her older, good-looking neighbor whom she had a crush on. Doing shit like that is totally counterproductive like a guy talking about getting dengue fever while he's on the Bataan death march. In addition to making me jealous, she was also good with the over-analysis

So, Where's My Girlfriend?

as she used to blow a fuse over the most trivial things. For example:

Me: *"You know that Batman is my favorite comic book hero"*
Her: *"So, what are you saying? Does that mean that you consider me Robin? Robin's a guy. Do you think I look like a guy? It's because you think my shoulders are too wide, don't you? Robin's a horrible dresser too. You think I'm a horrible dresser, don't you?*
Me: *"Holy Crazy Girlfriend"*

As mentioned earlier, I believed that the abuse I was getting was good for me. I really think that this relationship really messed me up good as I still feel the aftershocks reverberate in my present life by my inability to maintain a relationship with another human being that's anything remotely meaningful.

So the relationship lasted a month and it was crappy for me since I was going through puberty at that time. Naturally, I wanted to some action from this girl but I never saw her. As well, I knew that the relationship was going to end soon and she wasn't that type of girl to give pity sex. So, similar to a guy looting a burning house, I wanted to take what I can and get the hell out of there.

I wanted to kiss her. So one day, I decided that I would do just that.

I decided to do the old "grab and smash" in the relationship and hopefully have a make-out session with this girl before time ran out. One fine afternoon, I went over to her house to watch some TV. Conveniently, her family was gone so we were left to our own devices.

We headed to her basement and we sat together on the couch watching Oprah. With nothing but carnal intentions in my head, I began to mentally psyche myself up for the big moment. I told myself: *"I'm going to reach over and kiss her. How hard is that?"* Doing something like this for the first time in my life was horrendously scary – firing a guy who just lost his wife to a car accident and his grandmother to the Lochness Monster seemed like an easier task than kissing this girl for the first time. I could feel my heart beating fast the more I thought about it so I began to talk myself out of it. The horny side of me was determined however to get some "honey" from the jar. Finally, I told myself that I was going to kiss her after I count to ten in my head. Keep in mind that throughout

So, Where's My Girlfriend?

all of this, we were still watching *Oprah*. So without further hesitation, I began the
countdown in my head:

10…Oprah returns from commercial.

9… *"Now, I'd like to welcome someone truly special to the show"*

8…Adorable little white kid comes out.

7…He sits down.

6… *"His name is Michael…"*

5… *"…and he wants to say something to the crowd"*

4… *"Michael…"*

3… *"…go ahead"*

2… *"Oprah…"*

1… *"I have cancer"*

Stop.

How am I supposed to kiss this girl now? There's a kid with cancer on TV.

How romantic is this? It's like having a honeymoon in Rwanda during the genocides.

So I sat there and did nothing.

In my head, I hastily retreated. Maybe if I wait it out, everything was going to be all right.

Finally, she changed the channel to a show that didn't have an adorable kid with a life

threatening illness. I regrouped and decided to give it a second shot.

I turned my head to my left and stalked my prey again as she kept watching TV. I began

my descent and my head slowly started to travel across the couch. Slowly, I could see her

face getting bigger as my head kept inching forward. My face kept slowly advancing

towards hers…here it is…closer…closer…

Thump.

That's the sound that happens when someone jabs his nose into his girlfriend's cheek.

Apparently, I got so worked up about the approach that I totally forgot that I had to stick

my lips out and kiss her. What I did was something resembling a nose jab into her cheek.

When I nose jabbed her, I realized what had happened but had no recourse to correct it. I

quickly retreated back to my side of the couch and acted like nothing happened hoping

So, Where's My Girlfriend?

that she would think it was somebody else…perhaps it was that horny leprechaun that lived between the crawl space of her basement.

I could tell by her tomato red face that she was embarrassed and she was probably thinking hard as to where she had left her pepper spray. At this moment, I felt that this might be an opportune time to leave, so I suggested that perhaps I should be going. Unsurprisingly, she agreed so I got out of there faster than White farmers in Zimbabwe. When I got into my car on her driveway, I recounted the events that just transpired and I began to laugh hysterically over the entire incident. As I pulled out of her driveway laughing like a wild man, I looked up at her window and saw her staring right at me in horror.

Love is such a joke.

Lessons Learned

How to Kiss – Looking back, I think that I made two big mistakes in my attempt to kiss Amanda. If you can look at the jumbo screen: The first mistake was that I over-thought the situation. As Crash Davis says in *Bull Durham*, "*Don't think, just throw.*" When I try and talk myself out of doing something, it usually means that I haven't gathered the sufficient guts to do what I intend to do. When I want to talk myself out of something, you'd be surprised how much creative excuses I can come up with. Usually, when people find themselves in this predicament, they either turn to drinking to loosen the nerves or pray for the Holy Spirit for divine intervention. Unfortunately for me, I was below the drinking age at that time and as usual, God wasn't there when I needed. Leave a guy with a lot of mother-induced neuroses alone with a girl and he's bound to fuck it up. Yes, I'm blaming my mom.

As well, maybe I shouldn't have gone down the countdown route in my head since I wasn't in the business of launching rockets – I was in the business of kissing a girl. Counting down only brings tension and anticipation, which is only good when you're trying to celebrate New Year's Eve or holding up your end of a suicide pact.

The second critical mistake I committed in this romantic fiasco is to kiss her meekly. Firstly, I snuck in a blindsided kiss thereby catching her off guard. This is the equivalent to a sucker punch. A man does not sucker punch another man nor does he sucker kiss a

So, Where's My Girlfriend?

woman. The manly way to kiss a girl is to approach her directly thereby making his intentions clear:

Woman, here I am - clearly in front of you and my head is approaching yours. No, there is no magnet planted in my head that's forcing my head towards yours. I am clearly interested in engaging in this act of affection you humans have aptly called 'kissing'. If you don't reciprocate, I may take a vow of chastity. Now give in to me or my masculinity will go down faster than this erection I currently have.

Now, that is the manly way of doing it - quite direct and forceful. I've tried it both ways and I must say that the second one is so much more effective.

What Do I Have To Lose? – To this day, I do this and I don't know whether or not it's right: If I know that I have no intentions of having something serious with a girl, I'll still try and get something from her. It's like being down by 30 points in basketball with five seconds to go in the game and launching a three point shot just to pad your stats. This is clearly selfish but at the same time, won't affect the outcome of the game. When I realized that I was no longer interested in this girl is when I decided to milk it for all it's worth. Kind of an asshole move, I know – like taking a dead guy's wallet. Maybe I'm a petty guy. I also think that it has to do with my peers. Among guys, getting something from the girl, (whether it be a make-out session, a hand job or a $200 loan you don't intend to pay back) is a badge of honor. Guys pride themselves on their womanizing skills therefore no guy wants to be known as the one who invested all his time and effort into a girl, only to be denied everything but the exit. In this case, his guy friends will think that he got played, not the girl. Here's the big catch: it doesn't really matter if something did or didn't happen between the guy and the girl, all the guy cares about is what his buddies think. So, if you're a cool girl and don't really care what other guys think, help out your guy friend by telling his sorry-ass buddies that you two slept together and that he's a stallion in bed. I think a great illustration of my point comes from a scene in the movie: *Romi and Michelle's High School Reunion* (1997) when Mira Sorvino, in order to borrow a car, agrees to tell everyone at her workplace that she slept with the ugly mechanic who in turn, let her take the car.

Guys do it partly for respect among his guy friends. The other reason they do it is in a bid to impress other girls. You see, girls often use other girls as a benchmark/reference point in dating guys. When possible, a girl will check the track record of a guy by the girls he's dated to see if he's within her league. If a hot girl comes up on his "Girl's I've slept with" list, then his references have just checked out and he is now in line for a job from this new girl.

So, Where's My Girlfriend?

Not The College I Expected

When I first entered my freshman year of college, I was ready for some wild times. If movies like *Animal House* or *Van Wilder* were accurate portrayals of college life, then I couldn't help but hold some assumptions of how student life was going to be like once I hit college: co-eds, bra parties, excessive drinking and excessive sex. So, allow me to demonstrate the big chasm that separates Hollywood's idea of the student life with the reality of my student life.

This all began in Spanish class, my first class in my college life. Believing that Spanish people were going to take over the world, I thought it safe to start thinking ahead and learn the language of our future masters. (Unfortunately, my prediction appeared to be wrong – Chinese people will become our masters). So there I was, in the first class of my college career, I listened to my professor talk about Ricky Martin and all things Spanish. Bored, I scanned the room in search of any cute girls that might inhabit the same classroom as me. I quickly spotted this cute girl in front of me and I proceeded to give her the stalker glare. There she was, wearing a gray tank top and black pants, writing in her notebook. As she's writing, she dropped her pen on the floor and proceeded to bend over to pick it up. That's when I caught a glimpse of what every guy wants to see on a girl – a tattoo right above her bum. By picking up her pen, this girl quickly scored points in my book for being a possible "freak", (which I was promised to encounter throughout my student life as depicted by the Hollywood movies). Overjoyed by my visual discovery, I quickly turned to my right and made eye contact with a fellow male classmate who sat a seat apart from me. He gave me the smile and the "nod" which indicated that he also partakes in the act of creepily staring at girls in Spanish class. Class was eventually dismissed but not before the professor assigned us to small tutorial groups. Lo and behold, I found myself in the same group as my tattoo princess.

Within a short period of time, I got to know her quickly and found out that her name was Elizabeth. She was from out of town and therefore she lived alone on campus. Again, the revelation that this girl lived by herself was bonus points to my ear, as the possibility of 2am drunken booty calls raged restlessly in my mind so I quickly tried hard to become her friend.

So, Where's My Girlfriend?

One day, after class, Elizabeth and I had some time to kill before lunch. We were
casually walking back to the main campus when she turned to me and said,
"Do you want to go back to my residence?"
I quickly said yes since I was pretty sure she was going to sleep with me. Why else would
she ask me back to her residence?
With that, I marched triumphantly towards her residence. We entered her building and
got on the elevator and I couldn't press the "Close Door" button any faster. I think I shut
the door on a guy on crutches. In my head, the promise of some campus shagging
weighed heavily on my mind as I tried hard not to let my excitement show through the
physical manifestation of an erection.
I managed to keep my cool and finally, we reached her floor and entered her room. I
stepped inside and surveyed her room: just like any other student dormitory, it was a
mess. Clothes were strewn everywhere and empty pizza boxes lay on top of tables. I
didn't mind the mess since I figured I've never had sex on a pizza box before. So I
entered and sat down, waiting for the festivities to begin.
After five minutes of nothing, that's when I realized something critical. Something that
didn't hit me until the last second: I realized that I had no moves.
The Hollywood movies failed me in the sense that the girls typically threw themselves at
the guy. How come Elizabeth wasn't asking me to rub her back with oil? How come she
didn't want to voluntarily show off her bikini collection to me? Where was the pillow
fight between her and her friends? More importantly, why is Elizabeth taking out her
laptop? Well, I soon knew the answer when I discovered the bitter truth as to why I was
brought into her residence. With her laptop out, Elizabeth said:
*"By the way, I can't seem to get the battery out of this laptop, do you know how to do
it?"*
Thinking this was a test before she took in my manhood, I jumped at the chance to show
her my expertise in the art of taking out a laptop battery. Unfortunately, despite trying
repeatedly I couldn't take out that fucking battery. At that point, my fingers were sore
from trying (but I wasn't concerned as I was confident I could still use them on her).
After my futile attempt to take out that battery, I apologized and gave it back to her.
Then I said…

So, Where's My Girlfriend?

"So..."

She replied: *"So...are you hungry? Let's go eat!"*

With that, we went downstairs to her building and ate lunch at the cafeteria. To add insult to injury, I didn't have any money for lunch so she paid for me. I believe that she had my balls for lunch that day.

Lessons Learned

Porn is bad for you –When religious people tell you that porn is bad for you, they don't mean that you're going to die from watching it. Sure, you might burn in Hell for watching barely legal debutantes take it from all sides but porn isn't going to give you hairy palms or a third arm. I think porn is bad in the sense that it warps your mind into thinking that every situation is merely a build up to an eventual money shot. It's the psychological effect of Priming – when an earlier stimulus affects the response to a later stimulus (like me watching a porn on University co-eds before I go to lecture) it might cloud your judgment and expectations just a little. I confess that I am a big fan of the pornographic genre. In addition to Hollywood classics such as *Animal House* and *Van Wilder*, I also appreciate the cinematography of movies like *Kelly the Co-ed* and *Fast times at Deep Crack High*. As a result, I've been disappointed in a lot of instances when a girl doesn't put the whip cream on herself, instead of putting it on the apple pie. If you watch a lot of porn, you really begin to develop assumptions that any situation can turn into a threesome. Then again, I don't think that porn warps the mind to the extent that people are going to start driving around town without any pants. It just distorts reality in minor ways, like thinking that the girl is about to put out, but in actuality, she just wants her laptop battery taken out.

Wrong clues Sherlock – I have to confess that one of the reasons I thought that this girl was going to sleep with me was because she had a tattoo. I think that only sailors and "loose women" have tattoos. Clearly, I should quantum leap back to the early twentieth century. When I saw Elizabeth with her tattoo, the first thing I thought was: "Awesome, target practice!" Clearly, if she can do something as crazy as getting something permanently inked on her body, then she would easily do something not as crazy like sleep with that guy from Spanish class.

At that time (I don't feel the same today as I don't really care anymore), I felt that girls with tattoos were hot but were never marriage material since I could never take them home to meet mother. They were too much of a "bad girl" for my household

Being girlfriend material is fine but when it came time to play for keeps, I think most guys would prefer a fresh canvas over one that's already been inked.

Note: guys are picky and guys are assholes. Guys are picky assholes.

Living-at-home mentality vs. living-by-yourself – I think a big reason which escalated my misled belief that I was getting some easy sex from Elizabeth was her suggestion that we hang out in her residence. I went through my entire college experience living at home with my parents. People who have always lived at home have never felt the independence of living by themselves. So once they get that opportunity, it's like releasing a hungry animal out of its cage – the first thing it wants to do is to eat everything it sees. Once people begin to live by themselves however they quickly get over the initial novelty of independent living and soon, they're no longer hungry. I'm sure that the first time Elizabeth lived by herself on campus, she did everything she wasn't allowed to do when she was at home but she quickly got over it. For me however, the prospect of heading over to her residence and do something without the chance of mom hearing through the ventilation system was too good for me to bear.

Note to self: move out of mother's basement.

So, Where's My Girlfriend?

Better Left to the Professionals

I hope this story serves as a lesson to all the guys out there who think that they can date any type of girl. This story is for that librarian who thinks he can tame a stripper or the engineer who wants to date a beatnik poet.

I met Mandy at a club through a mutual acquaintance. Mandy was an attractive girl: she was petite and stood about 5'4" with straight shoulder length jet-black hair. She had pale skin which she emphasized with dark eye shadow and bright lipstick thereby making her look like a haute couture vampire. She would have been perfect as an extra in the *Blade* movie series.

When I met her, I knew to play it cool and acted nonchalant so I just made small talk whenever I ran into her that night. As the night progressed, I kept the drinks coming. Eventually, I had too much to drink and pretty much got wasted. I stopped remembering conversations I had with Mandy and just kept on nodding. More importantly, I was too drunk to remember giving my number out to her.

Well, a month later, I was quickly reminded when I got a phone call.

Here is how the conversation went:

Me: *"Hello?"*

Her: *"Hey, its me!"*

Me: (Thinking: Who the hell is this?) *"Uh…hey!"*

Her: *"So, how's it going?"*

Me: (At this point, I was drawing a blank so I decided to start asking questions in order to draw clues) *"So, are you just coming back from…school? Work?"*

Her: *"Oh, I just came back from school."*

Me: (Furiously going through my mental rolodex of all the barely legal girls I knew) *"Oh, I forgot, do you live downtown?"*

Her: *"Yeah…so what's new?"*

Me: *"Just chilling I guess, you know…"*

Her: *"Do you know who this is?"*

So, Where's My Girlfriend?

Me: *"Uh...Do you want to help me out here?"* (Note: I felt like an ass)
Her: *"It's Mandy!"*

After fifteen minutes of inane conversation and Mandy's overuse of the term
"like...yeah" I found out that Mandy was cordially inviting me to a birthday party of her
good friend at a club that coming weekend. Seeing how I was going to be at an early
party that same night near the area, I agreed.

So the weekend rolled around and I attend the first party. Throughout the night, I
received a steady stream of text messages from Mandy asking when I was going to make
my appearance at her party. I played it cool and gave her ambiguous Oracle-like answers
like *"I'll get there when the skies unite."* Finally, after her text began to look like she was
conceding defeat, I felt bad so I decided to get my friend, Cowboy to go with me to
Mandy's party. I looked good in front of my friends when I showed them Mandy's texts
and said, *"I have to go. This girl wants me so bad".*

(If this opportunity were to arise again, I would heavily recommend resisting the
temptation to giggle like a schoolgirl while simulating pelvic thrusts into the air.)

I proceeded to give Mandy a call and told her that I was on my way. The prospect of me
coming to see her excited her as much as the prospect of finding oil excites eighty year-
old Texans: Greatly. At this point, I figured that if I left my good friend's birthday party
just to see Mandy, she should at least let me get in the club for free. Cowboy and I made
an agreement that if we had to pay cover at Mandy's party, we would go back to my
other friend's party. Mandy assured me that Cowboy and I would get in for free so we
jumped into a taxi and got to the club. In a few minutes, we arrived at the club and
approached the bouncers. We gave them Mandy's name.

No dice.

The bouncers insisted that we pay for cover.

I texted Mandy: *"Bouncers won't let us in".*

I quickly received a text back instructing me to wait for her.

Within 30 seconds, she came flying out of the club to talk to the bouncers.

So, Where's My Girlfriend?

When she came out of the club, she was literally wearing lingerie and heels. It's like she forgot to put on clothes that night and went to the club thinking it was her bedroom. Anyway, she worked her magic and before we knew it, we walked into the club hassle and cover free. Not bad. We reached the dance floor and Cowboy and I met an assortment of Mandy's friends - each more scantily clad than the next though Mandy still took the cake.

Eager to be a good host, she asked if I wanted anything to drink.

I said, *"Whatever. Don't worry about it"*

She said, *"No, I'll get you a drink. Wait right here"*

At this point, she left and walked across the club where she proceeded to approach a group of guys standing by the bar. She began to talk to one of them and eventually convinced that guy to buy her a drink. She grabbed the drink and proceeded to walk it back and hand it to me. So pretty much what just happened was that this girl just hustled to get me a drink.

So the night continued on and Mandy would dance wildly around the club, then dance wildly up on me followed by dancing wildly with her friends. Safe to say, there was a lot of wild dancing going on. Throughout the night, Cowboy was busy talking to Mandy's friends and asking questions. Later that night, he pulled me aside and pointed to a fat guy looking at us from across the club.

Cowboy: *"You see that guy?"*
Me: *"Yeah."*
Cowboy: *"Do you know who that is?"*
Me: *"No."*
Cowboy: *"That's Mandy's date."*

I felt bad. I really did. Unless this guy got off watching his date accommodate other men (like that porno *Screw my wife, Please!* which my non-existent friend tells me about...) I'm sure the fat guy wasn't happy at all. At that point, I felt like the proverbial "bad guy" – the guy who finished first while the nice guy staggers in last place. I hate to say it, but

So, Where's My Girlfriend?

at the same time, it felt good to finish ahead of this guy. I felt like the Alpha Male in the room, which gave me a big power trip and made me want to high five people.

At this point, because it was a crappy club patronized by the riff-raff of society, a fight conveniently broke out in front of me. This fight comprised of a large, muscular guy beating a skinny five-foot girl unconscious. If that didn't signal the end of the night, I don't know what would.

Dancing elephants?

As we lined up for our coats, Mandy, watching the fight, sighed to me:

Mandy: *"(Sigh) that's the most action I've seen all night"*

Me: *"Well, if you wanted action, all you had to do was say so."*

Mandy: *"Really?"*

Me: *"Yup, it's that easy."* (Sounding like a spokesperson for an infomercial)

Mandy: *"Okay."*

Wow. I can't believe that worked.

I was totally caught off guard with her response as I find it rather difficult for girls to fess up to wanting sex. I simply asked it as a shot in the dark and I nailed it right on the head.

Well, I couldn't take her home that night because she had the fat guy looking after her. Instead, I got her MSN messenger information and her phone number (again) and bid her good night.

Sounds good right? Witness as I quickly turn from a hero to a zero in a matter of moments as the saga continues...

So, Where's My Girlfriend?

Better Left to the Professionals (Part 2)

I believe that somewhere in the Bible under Genesis, it mentioned that the Lord created
Monday for the purpose of contacting people you met on Friday. So, being a God-fearing
man, I promptly added Mandy to my MSN messenger on Monday and began having a
civil online conversation with her. I guess a big motivation I had in engaging her in some
discourse is to know some things about her. Things that might come in handy, such as:
What's her last name?
Where does she live?
Is she of legal age?

Here's how our conversation went:

Me: "*Hey*"
Her: "*Hey*"
Me: "*So, how was the rest of your Friday night…blah blah blah*"
Her: "blah blah blah"
Me: "*Good. So, yeah, when you're not busy with school, we should totally hang out.*"
Her: "*Can I ask you a question?*"
Me: "*Sure*"
Her: "*Are you gay?*"
Me: "*Gay?*"
Her: "*Yeah…are you gay?*"
Me: "*No. What makes you think that I'm gay?*"
Her: "*I don't know, you're so smiley and energetic.*"
Me: "*Well, I'm not gay. Is this a problem?*"
Her: "*Kind of. I think gay guys are so hot. I only sleep with gay guys.*"
Me: "*Okay, how does that make sense? Isn't the fact that they're gay kind of defeat the
purpose of them sleeping with you?*"
Her: "*I don't know. It's just something I'm obsessed with. One time, I had sex with a gay
guy and it was great.*"

So, Where's My Girlfriend?

Me: *"Well, if he had sex with you, I doubt that he's gay."*
Her: *"No, he was high on ecstasy and he thought I was a guy the entire time."*
Me: *"How so?"*
Her: *"He kept asking me where my penis was."*
Me: *"Oh."*

After this conversation (which was probably more bizarre than an interview with Charles Manson), I decided that it was best to end things. For reasons I'm sure is understandable to the reader, I felt that it was probably better for me to cut this dialogue early before the inmates got hold of the keys. Then again, there was a side in me that wanted to probe even further just to see where this would lead. Finally however, I logged off and decided that she was better left to the professionals.

<u>Lessons Learned</u>

Stay within your own league – Birds of a feather flock together. In other words, crazy-ass girls should hang out with crazy-ass guys. Perhaps I was too nice or too shocked to deal with it but I'm sure if I were wild, I would have had the right responses to this girl and got to plow her like a rural farm boy to his field in India. Perhaps, if I were crazy enough, I would have suggested recreating the ecstasy addled sex romp she had with the gay guy (with me playing the gay guy by talking with a lisp).

Unfortunately, this type of thing is usually out of bounds for me. Call me crazy but I would prefer playing the role of a heterosexual male in a sexual relationship. People should play within their own boundaries and not wander over to their neighbor's yard. It's not that I can't get a crazy girl-I probably can, but the question is: how long can I hold onto that bucking bronco before she throws me off or have me arrested with her crazy antics?

I think a good way to know your limits is to visit a strip club and have a conversation with a stripper. Whenever I'm in a strip club, I always end up engaging in conversations with the strippers. The things most of these strippers go through are pretty crazy. For example, one stripper was telling me that she didn't get along with her manager so one day, he locked her in a walk-in freezer and when she finally got out, she threw water in

So, Where's My Girlfriend?

his face (which I kind of got suspicious about since water would technically freeze in the freezer. I don't get stripper science) Anyway, stripper stories makes you realize that people live in very different worlds. Before you go and date a crazy-ass girl, you should ask yourself: am I ready to deal with things like this?

Do I have a walk-in freezer I can lock her in when she misbehaves?

You get the point.

Never buy a girl a drink – Buying a drink for a girl is very iffy to me as there are plenty of arguments for and against it. Usually, arguments against buying a drink come from guys since guys are very weary of girls using them only for drinks. Guys buy drinks for girls for one reason and one reason alone: to get into the girl's pants. Why else would a guy spend his hard-earned money on a girl he just met? He can do this in two ways: the first way is to keep buying her drinks until she gets drunk and sleeps with him or the second way is to buy her drinks, get her attention, get her number and eventually sleep with her. Either way, all roads still lead to Rome.

Also, remember that you're at a club, a place where people want to meet other people. You'll probably realize that there's a higher likelihood of meeting girls who will sleep with you tonight compared to buying a drink for a girl during brunch on a Sunday morning. Nobody is fooling anybody here: people are looking to hook up and buying a drink is a signal.

At the same time, there's the girl's perspective to this – just as a guy buys a girl a drink with the intention of sleeping with her, girls are not stupid and know the game that's being played. As one girl says, "*A guy will come up to me and offer to buy me a drink. I know that he just wants to sleep with me so I'll let him buy me a drink. After he gets me a drink, I'll say thank you and walk away.*" There are no victims in this game as everyone is out for their own self-interest. If the girl wants to sleep with the guy, she'll take the drink. If she doesn't want to sleep with the guy, she may or may not take that drink. Whatever the scenario is, the guy looking for sex has to offer to buy the girl a drink regardless. This is why a lot of guys now preach the importance of not buying a girl a drink if they think she's out to use them. This would weed out the population of girls who

So, Where's My Girlfriend?

only use guys for free drinks; girls like my friend Mandy, who wanted someone to buy her a drink so that she can give it to her ambiguously gay friend – me.

So, Where's My Girlfriend?

You, Me and That Other Guy

Whenever someone begins a sentence with, *"So I met someone over the Internet…"* chances are, that person is either on the evening news regarding a murder or just got himself arrested for meeting a thirteen year old at a motel room. The bottom line is that meeting people over the Internet is like that alleyway you saw in Mexico: it's probably better if you don't go there. Allow me to relate my personal experience with meeting someone over the Internet. After hearing this, the reader would probably be convinced that the Internet is best used for Fantasy sports pools and watching porn to pass the time at work.

This story takes place just after my graduation from university. I was working full time as an office monkey and I was bored out of my mind. My job was repetitive and required the mental ability of an autistic goldfish. Safe to say, when my mind becomes idle, the devil comes out to play with sharp knives. One day, I decided to dabble in Internet dating just for the hell of it so I found a credible website and began filling out my profile. Without a care in the world, I uploaded my profile and waited patiently for a fish to bite. A few weeks passed and I began to wonder how it was possible convicted inmates in prison find love through correspondence while I'm languishing in suburbia. Finally, I log in one faithful afternoon and find the words I longed for:
"Hey…"
So I open the message and it was something generic like *"I saw your profile and I think you're cool."*
Whatever it was, I replied.
This online correspondence continued back and forth several times. I don't remember how the dialogue went but I guess it must have gone well enough to warrant a face-to-face meeting with this girl for a date.
So here was the plan: our first date consisted of watching the movie *Pirates of the Caribbean II* followed by dessert. I was feeling nervous that night as I drove to the girl's house and waited for her patiently, As seconds turned to minutes, doubts began to creep into my head as to how she would look. The problem with the Internet is that there's

33

So, Where's My Girlfriend?

nothing to rely on other than a picture. This is when someone talented in Photoshop can trick unsuspecting daters like me. Secretly, I was praying that she didn't have a glass eye. Finally, out she came, she was those girls who were small but still had baby fat on them, she looked younger than she really was especially since she was wearing grey American Eagle track pants with a blue baby t-shirt. She topped this off with flowery designed flip-flops. I was aware that it was summer at that time but I couldn't help but feel that she was taking things a bit too casual, especially on a first date. Nevertheless, I soldiered on and we went to watch the movie. During the movie, she started doing things that kind of bothered me like putting her feet on the chair in front of her. Despite my incredible urge to enforce social norms on my date by giving her a lecture about the deteriorating morals and decency of today's society, I bit my tongue and let her degrade her morals away. Hey, it was a first date. I cut slack.

Afterwards, we stuck to the plan and proceeded over for some coffee and dessert where we chatted about stuff like friends and places to eat. I didn't recall much about the conversation but I did recall that when I dropped her home, she wanted a second date.

Our second date comprised of going to a club where we were going to meet her other friends. Before this date, I had already consulted with my female friends and they had all agreed that this was my acid test – this girl was going to present me to her friends to see if they liked me or not. I was told by my girlfriends to behave and to treat all her friends well. So, as I entered the club I immediately asked, *"Where are your friends?"* She replied: *"Oh, he's coming"*

Excuse me?

"He"?

In an attempt not to look jealous or concerned, I casually inquired about this male friend. I hoped that he would be the nice guy who finishes last (since I just found out from the last story that I can beat these guys) so I prodded:

Me: *"So, how do you know this guy? High school friend?"*
Her: *"Oh, Clive? He's a friend of a friend. I've just known him for a month"*

So, Where's My Girlfriend?

At this point, I became more concerned as she only knew me for two weeks. Did this girl decide to make friends only a month ago?

Me: *"So how did you become friends with him?"*
Her: *"Oh, Clive and I have a lot in common. He lives in the area I want to live and he has a cool place"*

Uh oh. I don't have a cool place. I live with my parents.

Her: *"Oh, here he comes now!"*

In walks Clive, with two girls. I quickly sized him up and realized that he looked just like me: the hairstyle, body type and the clothes. I realized that I was going up against my uglier twin from another uglier dimension. I hoped that one of the two girls he came with was his girlfriend.

Me: *"Are any of those his girlfriend?"*
Her: *"No, they're just friends from University"*

Soon enough, the two girls disappeared somewhere in the club and I found myself fighting my evil twin for the attention of my date. The night was kind of weird in the sense that when I bought my date a drink Clive would also buy her a drink. Then he bought all of us a drink so I returned the favor and bought all of us a drink. At the end, we bought drinks for each other. It's like you're kind of competing but you're pretending you're not. Dating is a tough sport man.
Nevertheless, Clive may have won some drink skirmishes that night, but I eventually won the date battle as I left the club with my date. Just to put my extra stamp on her, I proceeded to have a fifteen-minute make-out session in the car with her as I dropped her off. She sure tasted like the drinks Clive bought her.

So, Where's My Girlfriend?

At this point, you're beginning to see how guys are: this whole thing was now bigger than this girl, I was competing with Clive and this girl was the prize we were fighting over. The pissing contest has begun.

Just when I thought Clive was a one-time special appearance, I began to see this guy regularly whenever I would go out with this girl. For example, he would show up and hang out with us when we were with her friends at the beach. He would also hang out with us when we attended street festivals and other date-related events. I quickly realized that this houseguest was here to stay and there were only two beds for three people. Someone had to go.

Well, I soon found out who had to check out of the house when she asked me to meet her one morning at the mall. It was now winter and Christmas was fast approaching. She called and asked me to meet her at the change room of a store so I could give my input on some dresses she wanted to buy. I quickly got down to the mall and went inside the store. As I turned the corner towards the dressing rooms, I ran into a familiar nemesis.

"Hello", I said.
"Hello" said Clive.
"So, where is she?" I inquired.
"In the change room", he pointed.

Soon enough, she came out of the change room in a dress and asked each one of us for our opinion. Being men, we gave her one word grunts and statements that don't really say anything like *"I guess"* or *"If it's good, it's good"*. After she was done, she lined up at the cashier, so I took the liberty and inquired about the unwanted houseguest:

Me: *"What's HE doing here?"*
Her: *"Oh, I asked him to visit me on his lunch break"*
Me: *"So shouldn't he be having his lunch instead…alone?"*
Her: *"Haha, we'll go eat with him at the food court!"*

So, Where's My Girlfriend?

True to her wishes, we paraded over to the food court: just me, her and our special friend.
We proceeded to garble down some fast food fries and hamburgers. Finally, after the
meal was over, she suggested that we walk the third wheel to the subway to see him off.
I would rather push him off but I guess we can't always get what we want right?
So we walked to the subway to see Clive off.
"Bye!" she said.
With that, she leaned over and they proceed to open mouth kiss in front of me.
I was shocked.
I didn't know what to do.
Was I supposed to make out with her as well in front of him?
At that point, I knew the battle was lost. Rather, I knew the battle wasn't worth fighting
for. This was a country whose people I did not want to govern simply because the
citizens were plum insane. Take your fucking prize.
That was the last time I saw her.
That was also the last time I met someone online.

Log off.

Lessons Learned

The Merchant of Venice – In Shakespeare's *The Merchant of Venice*, Portia is a wealthy
heiress that had suitors coming for her left, right and centre. Whether it's a guy or a girl,
it's normal to feel good when you have suitors fighting over you. This is what pretty
much happened in this story: I had to fight it out with Clive. The weird thing about this is
that usually if a girl has a number of suitors, she would be more discreet. She would see
Guy A on Saturday and see Guy B on Sunday. Girls know better than to put two guys
head to head as things might get violent. This girl was gutsy though and pretty much had
me and Clive meet and hang out with each other. In a way, this is more pragmatic and
simple for the guy rather than having him always guess how many other guys she's
seeing. The downside to this is that it can get a bit too heavy – guys are visual creatures
and to literally see the competition may fuck up their head. It's good to see the

So, Where's My Girlfriend?

competition if he comes out way below your expectations. It sucks if he comes out and he's taller and more muscular than you.

"Friend" is such a loose term – I believe that the word "friend" has pretty much lost its meaning these days as people often use the word to label others they might have a romantic interest in. When someone doesn't know where the relationship is going between him and a girl, he can always say, *"She's just a friend"* to buy some time. As well, if a guy is cheating on his girl and they get spotted at a restaurant by a shared acquaintance, his whore can always be introduced as *"just a friend"*. At the same time that the word "friend" can save one's ass, it can also put the same ass away. How many times have guys felt the deadly sting of the phrase *"I like you, but only as a friend"* from the girl they've loved since grade school? For girls, they can use that word as a form of diplomatic immunity to mess with a guy's head. Like asking him to be their *"pretend boyfriend"*, watch movies with him and go on holidays with – all on the understanding *"that's what friends do"*. Then they get all shocked and angry when the guy misreads the signals and take his dick out during dinner. So, the lesson in this case was that the girl screwed me over by using the "friend" label for the other guy. By hiding under the "friend" guise, I couldn't do anything about it. Anything I did that mildly seemed defensive would have surely elicited the following question from her, *"You don't trust me? I said that he's only a friend!"*

So, Where's My Girlfriend?

When 2 for 1 Is No Good…

In today's world, everybody is always on the go. Everyone likes to multi-task and make the most of their time. People are so obsessed with being efficient that it trickles down to their personal life. Internet dating was created so people could click through potential mates like entrees on a menu while speed dating promises a maximum number of dates in the smallest amount of time. If this is today's world, then I believe that I should be excused for the time I double booked two dates in one day.

If the saying, *"Fool me once, shame on you. Fool me twice, shame on me"* holds any water, then I should have the shit shamed out of me since I didn't learn my lesson the first time and got burned twice as a result. Here is the story:

I met Nicole through a mutual friend and coincidentally Nicole and I went to the same gym. I saw her frequently and we would have brief discussions on general things like current events, seventeenth century art and transvestite prostitutes on Jerry Springer. Nicole was a small girl at about 5'2, pale skin and long black hair. She had big round eyes and was very cute. She looked like a Japanese cartoon character. Eventually, Nicole invited me for coffee and I accepted. At the same time this was going on, I was also semi-dating Susan, whom I met earlier in the summer. At this point, you might think that I'm being a dick for seeing two girls at the same time but to my defense, it was summer and I was single. I never verbally committed to a monogamous relationship with any of the girls. The rule is: If nothing is said, then nothing is agreed upon. In fact, one time I asked Susan about the status of our relationship.

She merely shrugged, so I shrugged.

There you go.

Free to play with the other kids.

On a Saturday afternoon, I met up with Nicole for our coffee. It turned out that Nicole wasn't just looking for a friendly chat. After our brief coffee talk, she invited me to see her condominium, which was conveniently located just above the coffee shop. At first, I wasn't too sure of her intentions. As we got on the elevator to her floor I decided that I

So, Where's My Girlfriend?

wasn't in the mood for a rape charge so I decided to ask some questions. Nicole mentioned that she shared the place with a roommate so I casually inquired as to the whereabouts of her roommate. Once she emphasized that the roommate was gone for the afternoon, I couldn't help but feel that love was in the air, waiting for me inside that 5'2" frame of hers.

I was led in and shown the place. We proceeded to sit down on her couch where she started to take out an album of glamour photos and proceeded to do a quick show-and - tell of it. The glamour photos were so touched up that I couldn't recognize that it was her in the photos. She peppered me with questions as to whether I liked the photos and whether or not I found the girl in the photos to be attractive. Now, I believe that this is the critical juncture of this adventure as she was probably fishing for compliments on her physically attractiveness (I know girls get insecure about their looks and stuff like that). What I'm about to say is the honest truth – sometimes, I think I suffer from one of those brain disorders where one can't clearly recognize faces. Stated plainly, I'm horrible at recognizing faces. If I were the town sheriff, the crime rate would increase every year because I wouldn't be able to recognize the bad guys on the wanted poster.

So, we now have a situation where I had a girl eager to show me glamour pictures of herself, while I'm sitting there asking myself why this girl is so obsessed with pictures of some other girl.

Being the modern day Sherlock Holmes, I quickly inferred that Nicole wanted assurance from me that she was the prettiest girl in the room. I had thought that the girl in the picture was some other girl and Nicole was looking for me to say that she was much more attractive than the girl in the picture. Perhaps this girl in the picture was Nicole's arch-nemesis? Then again, I don't remember Sherlock Holmes carrying glamour photos of Moriarty. Perhaps there's no nemesis. Perhaps the girl in the picture is actually Nicole.

Nicole: *"Do you think this girl in the picture is good looking?"*
Me: *"No"*
Nicole: *"No?"*
Me: *"Yeah, not good looking at all"*

So, Where's My Girlfriend?

Nicole: *"That's me!"*
Me: *(realizing that I'm fucked)* *"Uh...."*

At this point, I was completely caught-off guard and busted. As the parentheses indicated, I was fucked.
Quickly, I began to think about a way to save my ass.

Me: *"I mean I know it's you, I'm just saying that I like you better all natural. I like you right now"*

Whew.
I guess that line must have somehow worked because she didn't call security on me. She put the album away and turned to me. With her hand on my shoulder, she said *"So..."*
I began to slowly realize that there was a chance I was going to be in heavy make-out action with her that afternoon. I quickly looked at my watch – it was 4:15 pm.
Gah.
You see, thinking that coffee was going to be something quick, I had only allotted an hour in between seeing Nicole and Susan. Now, I was scheduled to see Susan at my house in half an hour. I knew that I could only stretch this out only for another 15 minutes. Instead of starting something and not finishing it, I decided that it was better to play hard to get in order to leave her wanting more so I blew Nicole off.
She was disappointed.
I proceeded to see Susan and we had dinner.
If I had known earlier that I could have gotten dessert from Nicole before dinner with Susan then I would have obviously managed my time better. I attribute this failure to poor scheduling on my part.
It turns out, I still didn't learn my lesson:

The second time I made a double booking, the situation was reversed where I was spending time with Susan and I had expected to see Nicole later on. I don't know why, but I always underestimate how far things might go on a date with a girl. Basically, I

So, Where's My Girlfriend?

planned to spend the entire Sunday with Susan, which I did. Again, I hadn't anticipated any special desserts afterwards. We spent the day at a festival eating and walking around – nothing too eventful. I've been taking it slow with Susan so I wasn't expecting anything other than a hug after the date. Thinking ahead, I began sending text messages to Nicole on my way home to find out what she was up to tonight since I had counted Susan out. There are two people you should never count out: Rocky Balboa and Susan.

Nicole was at a wedding and she was bored out of her mind. I kept trying to convince her to bail on the wedding and come visit me at home. She said that she'd think about it. Finally, Susan and I arrived back at my place. I was about to get out the car when she asked for something to drink.

Ever the gracious host, I proceeded to give her a glass of water. One thing led to another and before I knew it, we were engaged in some heavy make-out action. So, there we were, getting frisky on my couch when my phone tells me I have a text message.

"I'm coming over"
- Nicole

Fuck.

At this point, Susan gets so frisky that she's taken off my pants and she's on her knees. I began to quickly weigh my options:

Option A: Short-term gain – long term masturbation
- If I give Susan what she wants (namely, my manhood), there's a big chance that Nicole will ring my door and I'm literally caught with my pants down. I would have probably lost both girls the same night and they would have gone home together and engaged in some hardcore lesbian action without me.

Option B: Live to fight another day
- If I kick Susan out (in a gentlemanly fashion, of course) and wait for Nicole, I have a chance of scoring with Nicole. I reasoned that if I had gone this far with Susan

already, I should be able to go this far again the next time. By playing it safe, I get to be greedy and keep both girls.

I chose Option B.

I told Susan that I felt this was going too fast and she needed to go home. I waited for Nicole. She fucking never showed up.

Eventually, Nicole and I drifted apart and I never got my dessert. Susan eventually went away too, so I was left with nothing but excessive masturbation. Perhaps next time, I can spread my masturbation times an hour apart so that the left hand doesn't catch me with my right hand.

Lessons Learned

Those kind of girls – Some girls, like Nicole, never do what they say. I'm actually going through this with a girl right now - some people are just bad at doing what they say. Call it laziness or disinterest but some people need prodding just to get things moving. I knew a girl whose turn around time for texting was one day. If you texted her regarding dinner plans for tonight, she'd text back the next morning. I don't know how these people operate in this world. They probably get their electricity turned off every month because they're always behind on the bill payments. I'm upset at Nicole for not showing up that night. Had I known earlier what kind of girl Nicole was, I would never have kicked Susan out. So, the lesson here is to know what kind of girl you're dealing with. At the same time, if you looked at it from Nicole's perspective, she probably knew what was waiting for her had she come over to my house at night. She probably knew I was looking for some action and she didn't feel like giving it. Despite all the games guys play, I think most girls know when a guy is playing around. Guys are not details oriented and are sloppy which is why girls can always read a guy's intentions by the little hints he unknowingly gives out. The funny part though is that even if a girl has all the evidence in the world that the guy's not good for her, she will still go against reason and do what she feels like. She will talk to all her girlfriends to over analyze the situation in order to come

So, Where's My Girlfriend?

up with a conclusion to her liking. He can call her glamour shots unattractive and she'll still like him…or leave him hanging as a form of revenge.

Never Double-book – Double booking is all about being greedy and hedging your bets. I highly recommend against it. Aside from the obvious inconvenience of rushing from one place to another, guys also double book to feel good about themselves: that they're such a lady's man that they have to schedule seeing girls. This is bad though as double booking actually fucks up a guy's game as he'll be forced to put the moves quickly on a girl. As experienced guys know, girls like it when guys take their time. Unless the girl is looking for a straight booty call, you need to give her your time and attention because girls want to spend quality time with guys. Guys are pragmatic creatures and we have a hard time understanding this. Our rationale is simple:

Since you're going to dinner with me, clearly you like me. Since I asked you out to dinner, I like you. If we like each other, it's inevitable that we're going to have sex so we might as well save time by having sex now. By the way, why did you order the appetizer if you were only going to take three bites out of it?

If you do double book, never tell a girl that you double book since it's one of the biggest turn offs out there. Girls want to slap you for it. The reason is simple: put yourself in her shoes and imagine how you'd feel if a girl you're dating tells you that she's seeing another guy later after you. At the same time, double booking tells everyone that you're a player –which any girl over 18 is usually weary about. If you were a real player, you would know that it's all about showing a girl that you're not a player. Get it?

Evil guy trick technology update: As a result of the mass texting feature on cell phones, double booking has become easier to do. A lot of guys use the feature and create a list of all the girls he's currently talking to. He'll create a generic line such as: "*Hey, what are you up to tonight?*" or "*Hey, wanna hang out?*" then he'll hit send and wait. Soon, all the responses from all the girls will come pouring in and judging on the activities and availability, he can double book with the girl that best fits the schedule. I knew phone companies were evil.

So, Where's My Girlfriend?

The Things Your Friends Do…

This story is about my classmates giving me a helping hand during a university retreat over the winter, where we all stayed at a big chalet. The weekend consisted of boozing, partying and dancing. It was safe to say that there was going to be some other late night "activities" going on as well. Well, I certainly had this in mind and so did every other guy.

I was one of the first people to arrive at the chalet and that's when I first met Tamia. I saw her entering the chalet trying to haul her big suitcase so, being the gentleman that I think I am, I offered to lug it upstairs for her. When we reached her room, I placed her bag inside. She was about 5'6, skinny with a tanned complexion. She had these piercing dark brown eyes that felt like the type that always knew what you were thinking whenever she looked at you.

"Stay and have a beer with me!" she said.

Sure. What a cool chick.

There we were enjoying beers, when my friend, Crystal came in. Although the two girls didn't know each other, they were going to be sharing accommodations together.

I was happy since this meant that I now had a secret agent on the inside working for me. I quickly pulled Crystal aside and told her to play me up like I was an up and coming rapper that just got shot 18 times.

Crystal said *"Sure"*.

As the day progressed, I met more new people. I made friends and begin drinking. As day turned into night, everyone was drinking, dancing and being merry.

Tamia eventually wandered along and danced with me. Soon, she suggested that we relax in my room.

Now, at this point, I have to explain that my room was the default "party room" which was where the booze was kept. What this means is that, similar to a crackhouse, my room had a constant barrage of people going in and out. As the party slowly died down at around 3 am, there were four people left in my room. These people consisted of: Tamia, two guys and me. The two guys should have been clinically diseased from alcohol

So, Where's My Girlfriend?

poisoning yet somehow they were still functioning. At this point, I felt that it was time to start kicking out people who were not named Tamia as I wanted to make a move on her. Was she giving me signs? Maybe. To me, I considered the following cumulative things to warrant a green light:

- She had beers with me in her room.
- She danced with me the whole night.
- She was still in my room at 3 am.

In my country, that is sufficient evidence to warrant making a move on a girl. Looking back, these criteria seem a bit too lax and can definitely lead to miscommunication and inappropriate touching. I see how this can easily lead to a slippery slope: perhaps next time, if she makes eye contact with me means she wants it.

I hope guys that date rape don't read this book.

I guess I'm the type of person that tends to over-read a situation. I take any sign a girl gives as a welcome sign. This is the opposite of guys who are risk adverse: when girls throw signs their way, some guys prefer to err on the side of caution rather than risk being rejected by the girl. Luckily for me, I've done a fairly decent job reading the signs of the third base coach. So far, I haven't really totally misread a girl's signs. Stopped for going too fast? Several times, but stopped from driving in the first place? Never have.

I don't know – perhaps some girls are just too nice to say no. Perhaps some girls want to see how you kiss before she makes up her mind. Perhaps some girls say in their minds: *"About time!"* when you finally make your move. Whatever it is, I'm sure that I've missed more signs than I've misread. (**Note to self:** must learn how to read signs better and not rely on pornographic videos with simple sub-plots involving a strapping young prince and his flirtatious French maid.)

Whether or not Tamia was really giving the green light, I really wanted to make a move just to find out. I'm a risk taker like that – Gambling with your feelings is a lot cheaper than gambling with real money. It's almost cost-free (aside from the psychiatric bills I'll incur later in my life from years of womanizing that will probably cripple my ability to enjoy a meaningful relationship with women over nineteen).

So, Where's My Girlfriend?

The biggest challenge that faced me that night was trying to remove the two drunken guys in my room so I got up and tried to rush the guys out.

The first guy, although completely hammered, can see the ultimatum I offered in my eyes that either he left my room at that very moment or I was going to take his soul away. He quickly stumbled out.

The other guy however had no clue at all. He was determined to sit and watch TV until network cable ran out of shows. Unfortunately, Tamia got tired and announced that she was going back to her room. Upon hearing that Tamia was leaving, the drunken TV watching guy walked back with her. I was kind of suspicious that the drunken guy was trying to steal my dessert. I admit, I was paranoid that he was purposely blocking my game and now was trying to steal her away from me. I couldn't say anything however as I didn't want to look like the crazy guy so I kept my mouth shut. Whether it was truly cockblocking or a drunken personal foul, the bottom line was clear: That night, I slept with my pillows.

The next day, my friends begin pressing me for the details of my assumed debauchery from the previous night. Sure, I could have lied and could have told them that I went the distance with her, but I didn't because I don't like making things up. I'm not into starting rumours. Instead, I confessed my shortcomings that night and blamed it on the cockblocking by the drunken guy. My friends, so supportive towards my cause, decided to help me out. First, they approached the cockblocker and told him not to do it again on the threat of being labeled "The Official School Cockblocker". The guy personally apologized to me later in the day with a very heart felt: *"Hey man, I'm sorry I cockblocked you. I didn't know"*. Secondly, my friends pledged that they would do their best to leave me alone with Tamia when the time came.

The plan was set.

The activity for the second night was pretty much the same as the first – get smashed, dance and party away. Sometime during the night, I happened to run into my friend Crystal, my spy whom Tamia was sharing a room with.

I quickly pulled her aside and ask her for a quick debriefing about Tamia.

So, Where's My Girlfriend?

Crystal bluntly replies: *"She's only hanging around you because she thinks you're friendly and she doesn't know anyone else. I don't think you have a chance."*

This was a critical juncture: should I continue to invest in my time and effort with Tamia or should I take Crystal's advice and cut my losses? I decided not to listen to Crystal. Part of my reason for not listening to Crystal and to continue working on Tamia is because I felt that I had passed the point of no return. Out of the two and a half days we were going to spend together that weekend, I'd already spent a good day and a half with her, which meant that it would have been a waste to not see where this took me. It's like reading a book past the halfway point and then realizing that the plot has taken a ridiculous twist. Though you might be tempted to put the book down and read something else, you feel compelled to finish what you started just because of all the time you've already spent reading the damn thing (you're not at the halfway point of this book yet – I won't take offence). Then again, if I had cut myself loose from Tamia and looked for someone else, I might be guaranteed something more promising. For a second, I was really caught in the middle of the crossroads but then the dealbreaker came:
I realized that throughout the one and a half day I spent with Tamia, I was *seen* by everyone else spending time with her. This has two consequences: first, the other girls on the trip have associated me and Tamia together. This might discourage any other girls from flirting with me because they may think that:
  a) Tamia might get mad at them for "taking her man"
  b) They might look like "the other woman" and be labeled a slut
  c) They are just sloppy seconds
Plus, I realized, if I no longer pursued Tamia, I would look bad. It would look like I couldn't close the deal and she rejected me. My reputation was pretty much at stake.
As well, I was positive that she was giving the right signals to me and Crystal had just not seen it.
When night rolled around, the music and booze once again kicked in. The dancefloor was packed and again, the mating ritual began as I started to dance with Tamia. Before I knew it, we were grinding up on each other and taking pictures together.
Later on, she turned to me and says: *"Let's go hang out in your room."*

So, Where's My Girlfriend?

This is me getting another shot at it. Round 2.

We entered my room and once again it looked like a crackhouse with people passing out on the floor, pissing outside and having funnel wars (although I don't recall crack users using funnels). Upon seeing me enter with Tamia, my friends sprung into action and began to clear the room faster than a bomb threat at the White House. They began to shove people out of the room, taking drinks and putting them outside. Some people were literally grabbed and dragged away. Within two minutes, the place was cleared out, leaving only me and Tamia in the room. Pushing the last guy out the room, my friend turned to me, winked and then closed the door.

SLAM.

With that, Tamia's senses came about. She turned her head around and she quickly asked: *"Where did all the people go? Why is that door closed?"*

At that point, there was an awkward silence. With her asking those probing, innocent questions, I never felt like a bigger rapist than that particular moment.

When you're in a situation where the room is empty and the girl is wondering why, you really can't do or say anything that doesn't qualify as creepy. I wasn't going to make any moves.

"Open the door" she commanded.

So I did.

And the people came flooding back. My friends came back in and looked at me for a response. I could only look back in shame…

As the night slowly died out, people began retiring back to their rooms. Once again, I found myself with Tamia back in my room but this time, my roommate was also there. Apparently, someone had passed out in my bed so I had to sleep on the couch but the couch smelled like ass and beer so Tamia suggests: *"Why don't you sleep in my room?"*

What a brilliant idea - Why don't I sleep in your room?

Again, I ask: are these not signals?

At that point, I felt that I had finally hit the jackpot. This time, there were to be no drunken cockblockers. It was a direct but at the same time, indirect way to ask me to her room. How convenient: I had no place to sleep for the night.

So, Where's My Girlfriend?

So, we proceeded to head up to her room with thoughts of erotic ecstasy dancing in my head. As we entered the room, we suddenly saw my friend Crystal talking to a friend. Upon seeing my grand entrance, Crystal grabbed our friend and rushed out the door to leave us alone. Throughout the entire ordeal, I felt like we had the bubonic plague as wherever Tamia and I went, people would clear out. Tamia began to fix up the couch for me. She told me that she needed to use the bathroom for a second.

I eagerly wait by sitting on the bed. Then, I felt like lying down a bit because it felt so good and I was so tired…whoa…this bed felt so good.

I was so tired and this bed felt really good.

This bed felt really good…

This bed felt really good on my tired body.

I pass out.

When I woke up, it was the next day.

FUCK.

Lesson Learned

Always Listen To Girls – If I had taken my friend Crystal's scouting report seriously, I would have saved myself a lot of time and possibly salvaged the weekend. Not listening to a girl about other girls is like gambling against the house in Vegas. The house always wins. Guys who trust their own instincts is like trying to find your way without a map while trusting a girl's instincts is like navigating with a GPS. Sometimes, guy instincts could be correct and they find their way out of the woods but most of the time guys are completely wrong and end up being a grizzly bear's bitch.

To reiterate, girls are useful allies when it comes to deciphering the mysterious, cryptic messages of the female gender. They're kind of like the Windtalkers in this war between men and women. The only thing to watch out for however is to make sure that the girl who's supposed to be helping you is actually on your side…and not working to sabotage you. So why would a girl want to sabotage your chances with another girl? Sometimes, it's because SHE actually likes you and wants to make sure no one else gets close to you. Other times, some girls are just fucked up. I know girls who feel that it's their duty to

So, Where's My Girlfriend?

make sure she picks the best possible female candidate for me. This means disqualifying a lot of girls on different grounds. For example, she'll say: "*Oh, you don't want this girl. She's no good for you. Don't settle for that*". Here is the difference between guys and girls: with a guy friend, he'll do all that he can to help you get the girl YOU WANT. Girls on the other hand, will do all that she can to help you get a girl SHE THINKS you should be with. This is like walking into an electronic store with the intention of buying a forty inch TV but instead of selling you the TV, the salesperson insists that you buy a projector instead. Sure, it might be better but that's not what you want. Can I just buy my TV and get the hell out of the store?

Don't Be Super Nice– When I was young, my parents always taught me to be nice, and to be polite to other people. When I was nice and polite, other people were polite to me. This formula doesn't seem to work when it comes to getting girls. Sure, being a perfect gentleman might work when you're on a date, but at some point, there has to be that exciting moment when the guy says: "Fuck this" and kisses the girl. That weekend, I couldn't find my guts to not be nice and make a direct move on Tamia. Nice guys do nice things. Most of the time, nice guys don't take the initiative to make a move on a girl because that would be imposing – and that wouldn't be a nice thing to do. Maybe the formalities and pleasantries would be necessary had I been dating her but I think given the circumstances and the situation we were in (aka: an alcohol fuelled retreat), the threshold to make a move on her allowed a bit leeway. I should have totally tried something and not fallen asleep like an idiot.

That kind of girl – To this day, I still wonder whether this girl was really into me or whether that was just her personality. Some girls in this world are just flirty towards every guy. That's just who they are. Are they doing it on purpose? Is this a subconscious thing? Who knows? Perhaps they get off on leading guys on? The bottom line is: it's quite possible that she's just being flirty with me, but she's not actually interested. A good way to see if a girl is flirty is to watch how she acts towards other guys. If she's only flirty to me, then she might like me, but if she's flirty towards the entire lacrosse team, perhaps she's just a flirty girl.

So, Where's My Girlfriend?

2 Stories on Dating Karma

Story 1: Knock around Girls

It was around 10pm on a cool Saturday evening during the fall and I was on my way to a lounge to meet some friends. All alone, I walked down the street and found the place. As I headed towards the door, two girls walked towards me. We all reached the door at the same time. As I grabbed the door for them, I asked:

"Do you guys know if this place has a cover charge?"

One girl laughed and said, *"I'm not sure, since it's my first time at this particular lounge."*

I replied, *"I guess we'll find out soon enough."*

Again, she laughed. Why was she laughing so much?

What I said wasn't even funny. I didn't mean it to be funny. I guess this is what humans call flirting: when girls laugh at things you say that aren't even funny. I was pretty sure that she was interested in me since no one laughs at shit like that.

In terms of looks, she was kind of a big girl. Not fat, but she had a few pounds on her. As well, her face was kind of round and she was pale. Let's just say that you can get away with drawing her face using only a compass and a protractor. She quickly introduced herself as Sally and during the brief moment we spent walking down the stairs, we got to know each other. I found out that Sally was an undergraduate student studying history and it was her friend's birthday. She found out that I had just recently finished my first year of graduate studies. Once we got to the bottom of the stairs however, I separated from her, as I needed to find my friends. As well, I didn't want to look like a loser who went to the lounge all by myself so I had to show her that my friends really did exist.

I proceeded to walk around the place and quickly found my friends. After saying hi, I realized that I was the only one without a drink in my hand. Never one to let injustice occur, I excused myself and headed over to the bar. I promptly got the bartender's attention and ordered a beer. As I paid him accordingly, Sally wandered over to the bar.

Sally: *"Hey"*

Me: *"Hey"*

So, Where's My Girlfriend?

Sally: *"So you found your friends huh?"*
Me: *"Yep and you found your birthday girl?"*
Sally: *"Yeah"*

(Silence)

At this point, I had a good opinion of Sally. She was friendly and a bit persistent. I liked that. Then, it all went downhill from there:

Sally: *"So…I know you're a struggling grad student and all but…do you want to buy me a drink?"*
Me: *"Uhhhh…not really…"*
Her: *"Why not?"*
Me: *"Why should I?"*
Her: *"How about this, I buy you a drink and you buy me a drink?"*
Me: *"Not really."*
Her: *"Why?"*
Me: *"Because I'm already holding a drink"* (showing her my beer)
Her: *"I guess I'm not good at negotiating, huh?"*
Me: *"Apparently not, you can't seem to identify what my needs are"* (which is the principle of negotiating)

With that little exchange, we parted ways and she returned to her group while I returned to mine.

The End.

So, Where's My Girlfriend?

Story 2: Sex and the Wrong City

One time, my friends and I went to a club and we struck up a conversation with a group of girls. I started up a conversation with a cute girl with a killer smile and I asked her if she wanted to play this bar game I recently learned. She agreed and we began to play. So we made a wager which was: *The loser of the game had to buy the winner a drink.*

Lo and behold, this girl turned out to be a smart cookie and she beat me at my own game. I told her that she won fair and square and I was going to get her a drink.

So I asked: *"Shall we head for the bar now?"*

"Wait" she commanded. *"I need to get my girls"*

"Why?" I innocently inquired.

"Because I want to know what they all want to drink" she replied.

"That's nice. You're getting a drink for your friends" I interjected.

"No, you're getting a drink for all of us" she commanded.

Hahaha....No.

This, fellow readers...is called *The Shit Test.*

This is a zero sum game where you either pass or fail. This is the moment of truth where either a guy stands up as a man or he hands over his manliness to her in exchange for a lifetime of servitude to her. If he fails this test, he might as well assume the fetal position. To me, I felt that it was a slippery slope: Today, I'm buying drinks for her friends. Tomorrow, she'll have me building the pyramids.

So it was safe to assume that I was adamant that there was no way in bloody hell I was going to feed her army of darkness. First, I tried to refer to the terms of our agreement:

"The bet was one drink for the winner. That's one person."

She countered by repetition:

"No. You're buying for all of us."

I counter by inquisition:

"Why, may I ask do I need to quench the thirst of thy underlings?"

Then she pulled out the line...

"In Sex and the City, the girls do everything together"

When she said that, I knew what kind of girl she was. Everything had been solved. She was just another girl who thought she was Carrie Bradshaw from *Sex and the City.*

So, Where's My Girlfriend?

I've encountered numerous girls who think they're Carrie Bradshaw. They think that they deserve Mr. Big treatment. As much as she'd enjoy the Mr. Big treatment, I'd like to point out several things:

- Carrie Bradshaw is a fictional character - in fact, Sarah Jessica Parker does not even have a "Mr. Big" in real life. She has...Matthew Broderick.
- Assessing her conversation and wit, the girl was more of a *Hannah Montana* type of girl than *Sex and the City*.

Undeterred, she kept pressing with her demands of drinks around the house.
I gave her one last chance:
"You're only entitled to one drink. Do you want this drink?"
Again, she replied:
"Only if my friends all get a drink."
So I replied:

"Then your friends all better take small sips"

With that I walked away.
I bet Carrie never got that line.

Lessons Learned

The Giving and the Taking – Rejection and failure will always be part of Life and this is especially prevalent in the cold world of dating. People who date are like pieces of a puzzle, going around trying to find out whether they fit with someone else. If the pieces don't fit, it's okay to say "too bad" and walk away. People who reject you don't know you so you can't take rejection personally. As well, people in the dating world like to play the role of the victim when they say shit like: *"Why can't I find someone nice?"* People tend to only remember the times they get rejected by someone else and not the times they rejected other people. It goes both ways – some days you get rejected and other days, you reject someone else. For that person, she just got rejected by you but next time, she might reject someone else. Dating is a contact sport – you should learn how to

So, Where's My Girlfriend?

give hits and you should also learn how to take hits. When you do get hit, know that it's part of the sport and nothing personal. If someone doesn't want to live with the possibility of being rejected, then he should get a dog since dogs will never reject their masters. If a dog ever rejects him, then he should get a goldfish. If a goldfish rejects him, he should flush it down the toilet. At the same time, there's also a difference between not taking rejection personally and learning from your rejection. There might be something you're doing that rubs people the wrong way, hence getting you rejected. Perhaps you're a close talker or perhaps you like to make jokes about incest – who knows? No one is perfect, especially in the dating world and getting constantly rejected might be an indicator that you might have some things you can work on. This is when people get testy and refuse to acknowledge weakness. You can always use the cop-out excuse that *"If she didn't want me for who I am, then I don't want her anyway"* but that's usually a shitty excuse to be lazy and avoid self-improvement. You can have a restaurant that serves the best food but if the place looks like a dump, nobody is going inside to eat. Be open to criticisms: just because getting hit is inevitable, it doesn't mean you can't minimize them.

Short Con vs. Long Con – If the girl in the first story just wanted to score a drink from me, she must have an opportunistic mentality to say, *"I bet I can score a drink off that guy I just met at the door".* Some girls play a Short-con game (as opposed to girls who play a Long-con game). A Short-con game is pretty much when a con artist rips someone off in one short time period. For example, those crooked card games people run on the sidewalks are examples of Short-con games. It's usually a one shot, one deal with a small reward. In that card game, the hustler probably rips off $10 from the victim and the entire process takes about 15 minutes.

This is similar to an opportunistic girl at a club: she might invest 15 minutes of her time talking to her victim. Once she gets a drink from him, he may never see her again for the rest of his life. From the girl's perspective, this is actually very shortsighted (as she only gets one drink).

What opportunistic girls need is to run Long-con games. A Long-con game is a scam that may take several days to several years and the reward is usually larger (given the large amount of effort put in it). For example, a pyramid scheme is a Long-con game. Con

So, Where's My Girlfriend?

artists would probably need to wine and dine investors several times before they make the decision to invest their money with the criminals. Obviously, there's so much more complexity and effort in it, but the payout would be huge if it works.

So, how does this apply to these girls? Well, the biggest mistake these girls make is to bail on the guy after the drink. This is the equivalent of leaving a well after one has just filled his bucket. Why won't she see how much water she can draw from this well before it runs dry? Opportunistic girls should consider staying with their victims and see where it goes. What if he wants to buy her dinner after the drink?

What if he wants to take her on a vacation?

What if she becomes accustomed to how he treats her and she slowly finds his stability to be attractive?

She's just gotten herself into a relationship.

At this point, it looks like she's the one that just got screwed.

Be always ready to walk away - Dealing with a girl is like someone spending their first day in prison – the other inmates are going to test him. His reaction will dictate his status throughout his incarceration. In order to pass the test, this poor guy needs to beat a tough guy senseless with his prison tray in the cafeteria.

If a girl tests a guy and he doesn't show her any boundaries, she'll lose all her respect for him. If these boots were made for walking, then she's going to walk all over him.

If a girl ever calls a guy out on what he says, he better be sure to always be ready to back it up. There's nothing sadder than a guy who says things then folds when challenged by the girl. As well, it makes him look like a man with principles if he does exactly what he said he'd do. Finally, it also made sense for me to walk away from the girl in the club since I didn't have enough money to buy all her friends a drink.

So, Where's My Girlfriend?

The Sex Clause Agreement

This story attempts to show how sex can be used as a bargaining chip for anything. If professional athletes read this, they'll demand a sex clause in their contract negotiations. If the sports agent has a pretty mouth, he better watch out.

I met Rosa at a friend's house party. She came with her best friend Sheila who, at that time was interested in my friend Rudy. That night, I played Rudy's wingman and eventually met Rosa. As logic would dictate, it was only a matter of time later that night when I befriended Rosa and eventually got her phone number. So this is what happened:

Rudy → Sheila
Me → Rosa

Rosa was a recent graduate in physiotherapy. She had a muscular build and her body was toned. She stood about 5'5 with long black hair. She spoke in a faint, girly tone that always had me straining just to hear her. She also didn't have much to say, which meant that she did the listening and only answered me when I asked a question, which kind of bothered me since I preferred girls that were a bit chatty and proactive. A good example of a conversation with her would go something like this:

Take One (with a regular person)
Me: "*So, I went downtown today looking to buy a cheesecake…*"
Regular Person would have said: "*Oh wow, cheesecake! Why did you go downtown to buy a cheesecake?*"
Me: "*I wanted to buy a cheesecake because its my grandmother's 100th birthday this Sunday and I'm planning on missing it to watch the football game while I eat the cheesecake.*"
Regular Person would have said: "*You cold-hearted bastard. How dare you skip your grandmother's centennial birthday in order to watch football with cheesecake. At least order a walnut cake!*"

So, Where's My Girlfriend?

Take Two (with Rosa)

Me: *"So, I went downtown today looking to buy a cheesecake…"*

Rosa: (silence)

Me: *"I wanted to buy a cheesecake because its my grandmother's 100th birthday this Sunday and I'm planning on missing it to watch the football game while I eat the cheesecake."*

Rosa: (silence)

Me: *"So…do you like cheesecake?"*

Her: *"Yeah, I guess…"*

Alas, always the one to give someone the benefit of the doubt, (and never to turn down a girl who can give free physiotherapy massages) I took her phone number and promised to call her. Eventually, I called her and we talked on the phone. Talking to her on the phone was more painful than having your leg amputated by a plastic knife. I didn't really feel any fireworks. Simply put: I didn't connect with this girl. We were simply on two different wavelengths. As a result, I didn't really try that hard to call her. However, because Rudy was still dating Sheila, I kept finding myself in Rosa's presence whenever I went out with Rudy. After a month of dating, things between Rudy and Sheila eventually went sour but that didn't seem to impact the relationship between Rosa and me. Perhaps it was my loneliness or perhaps it was out of sheer boredom but I continued to keep in contact with Rosa. Once in a while, I would send her a text message or call her out of the blue when I had nothing to do. It seemed to be something I did out of convenience, but she would always return my calls so I kept doing it.

Sometimes, I feel bad for stringing her along in something I wasn't really serious about but sometimes I wonder whether she was doing the same thing to me as well.

I soon found out one faithful day…

The build-up began when I agreed to meet up with Rosa after her night class. When I saw her, she told me that we were also meeting Sheila for dinner. Despite being caught off-guard with this news, I didn't mind since Sheila would probably add some substance to the painful tooth-extracting conversation I was anticipating with Rosa. So we met up with

So, Where's My Girlfriend?

Sheila and we went for dinner. During dinner, the three of us chatted about relationships. The topic soon moved to sex. I wondered loudly:

"Remember those times in high school when guys would propose casual sex to girls?"
They both shook their heads. Rosa said, *"That's never happened to me before."* Sheila followed, *"Neither has it to me but I can see myself trying it."*
Rosa added in, *"Me too."*
I quickly concluded two things from their response:

1) I went to a high school inhabited by perverts.
2) These two girls were willing to try casual sex.

Before anything inappropriate could be suggested out of my mouth, I had to make sure I heard correctly. I decided to probe a bit deeper.
Me: *"So what do you define as casual sex?"*
Sheila: *"Well, someone I wouldn't mind seeing casually. Someone to spend time, watch movies and sleeping with."*
Me: *"Essentially, you want a boyfriend."*
Rosa: *"No, I wouldn't need this person to be constantly with me. Just someone to see me casually."*
Me: *"Would you expect him to be exclusive to you?"*
Both: *"Yeah"*
Me: *"So let me get this straight, both of you define a casual sex partner as someone who will spend time with you, watch movies with you and sleep with you exclusively?"*
Both: *"Yes"*
Me: *"That's called a boyfriend."*

To this day, I'm curious as to what they would define an actual relationship to be if they defined a casual relationship to be essentially a monogamous relationship. I'm thinking something like the scene in Star Wars where Jabba the Hutt had Princess Leia in chains.

So, Where's My Girlfriend?

A week rolls by and one night, I went to a networking event with Rudy. Lo and behold, we find Sheila and Rosa at the same event. Thankfully, even though things went sour between Rudy and Sheila, they were still civil towards each other. At the end of the event, the four of us ended up going out for drinks at another bar. During drinks, Rosa began to play footsy with me. By the end of the night the flirting had escalated to the point where her leg was on top of mine. It was safe to say that she was "hitting" on me. Rudy was a good friend and noticed what was happening. He wanted to help me out so after the drinks, he suggested that we all take a walk on the nearby beach, as he's never seen the beach at midnight.

Perhaps Rudy truly wanted to observe the beauty of the beach in all its glory at midnight or perhaps he wanted to give me an opportunity to be frisky with this girl in the confines of a deserted area at midnight. So Rudy wanted to help me out and Rosa was giving me all the signs that she wanted to fool around. When all the arrows point one way, it's hard to go the opposite direction so I agreed and we all went to the beach.

Upon reaching the beach, we broke off into couples. Rudy walked with Sheila while I walked with my arm around Rosa. We walked a few paces when Rosa suddenly whispered to me:

"I want to sit down over there." (Pointing to a picnic table)
"Sure." I replied.

With that, I informed Rudy to go ahead as we were going to take in the view of the beach from the picnic table (since that's what people do at midnight at the beach). So Rosa and I headed to the picnic table, where I proceeded to sit and enjoy the view…of her chest. Apparently, Rosa didn't want to sit on the table, but wanted to straddle me instead. She was quick to pounce and engage in a make-out session with me.

Well, almost.

After a few kisses, Rosa pulled back and said: *"Why do you like me?"*

I was totally caught off-guard. I hate it when girls ask this question. My brain struggled hard to think of the magic words I needed to say to have her resuming what she was

So, Where's My Girlfriend?

doing. My first tendency was to say something totally inappropriate like *"I like you because you're straddling me like we're in the Kentucky Derby."*

Thankfully, I was able to hold back the smart-ass comments. However, I still needed to answer the lady's question or risk spending the night locked in my bathroom with a *GQ* of Jessica Simpson. Here was the best response I came up with:

"I like you because I think you're a cool and neat girl."

What a crappy answer.

Maybe not…apparently, the judges deemed this answer acceptable as she resumed making out with me like we were in a fifties drive-in theatre. After a few minutes, Rudy and Sheila returned so Rosa had to dismount me and we walked back to the car.

After that, I went home.

A week later, I got a call from Rosa. She wanted to meet up with me in the evening. That night, I met up with her and took her back to my place. We began fooling around again but this time, we were in my bed. Nothing was there to stop us – no Rudy, no Sheila, no beluga whales or the night watchman. No one…except her.

Again, Rosa abruptly stopped our make-out session just when I thought this movie would turn from PG to NC-17.

She wanted to talk.

What did she want to talk about? What else do girls want to talk about?

Us.

A relationship.

Well, not really – she wanted to talk about maintaining something like a casual sex relationship. The same one she eluded to a few days ago. I quickly recalled her definition of casual sex as essentially a monogamous relationship. I don't know where the "casual" fits in (Perhaps I was allowed to wear jogging pants and large t-shirts when I saw her). Still, I wanted to hear her out. First I asked why she didn't just want to have an open relationship. Her response was that she's already had that experience in the past and was no longer a fan of it. She didn't want the drama that usually accompanied it. I made it

So, Where's My Girlfriend?

clear that I wasn't in the market for a serious relationship. She made it clear that she was.
So how does this work? What was she proposing?

This was the proposal:

If I went out with her, I got anything I wanted sexually.

Rosa was apparently quite the kinky girl. She pretty much would let me have my way
with her and would let me indulge in whatever I wanted. She would even do a threesome.
In fact, she told me that when she was younger, she secretly wanted to be a porn star. Not
just a stripper, but a bona fide porn star. How did her career counseling sessions go in
high school?

As one can presume, when she was telling me these things, my imagination ran amok in
my head and killed my rationality with a broken shard of glass but then again, this sounds
too good to be true.

So, what was the catch? There's always a catch.

This was her catch: She wanted me to enter a monogamous relationship with her for a
minimum of three months. During those three months, I couldn't sleep with her.

When I thought about it, she was essentially using sex as a bargaining chip to entice me
into a relationship with her. I've never experienced this before as sex usually came hand
in hand with the relationship, like free glasses of water in a restaurant.

I inquired as to why it had to be three months. Why not two months? Why not one and a
half? Three months seemed a bit arbitrary. She had no rationale for it. She just thought
three months was a safe number - so there was the deal.

I tried to bargain and argue for something less than three months but she wouldn't budge.
She wouldn't compromise. I thought hard about this arrangement and realized that this
was set up to put me in a very vulnerable position. The first obvious drawback from her
arrangement was that I was at her mercy in regards to sex. Essentially, she got what she
wanted (i.e. a relationship) before I could get what I wanted (i.e. sex). What if, after three
months, she decided to break up with me? I would have been screwed (not literally,
unfortunately) since I invested all that time for something that never came to fruition.
Here is the concept of Opportunity Cost: If I invest three months of my life with Rosa,
that's three months I could have invested in another girl I may like more. As well, it can

also be possible that Rosa was just talking a big game in regards to her sexual habits in order for me to bite at her bait. What if after three months, she was very conservative? It would be ungentlemanly of me to force her into a threesome. Finally, I realized that if sex is the only thing that's enticing me into this relationship, then I'd probably be miserable for the first three months I'm with her. Even if I began sleeping with her after the three-month trial date expired, I'm not sure sex could keep me interested in the relationship. I felt kind of sad. Sure, there was a chance I could fall in love with her within the first three months but I'm not the type that eventually falls in love with someone. My gut instincts told me to abort the mission. It felt wrong and artificial even for someone as superficial as me. Finally, my decision to walk out of her contract was also out of spite. I felt that I had to punish her for her inability to compromise on any of the terms of contract she proposed.

Contract terminated.

Lessons Learned

Sure Thing – What would you do if I told you that there was a game out there where if you played, you would win every single time guaranteed? At first, you would probably be delighted and play just to see if this is true. After 197 consecutive wins however you'd probably get bored of it. The reason why people love watching sports and why we tolerate upsets in sports is because the possibility of losing gets us excited. Despite the stigma society has placed on losing, I think that deep down, people like losing once in a while because it gives them hope of doing better next time. Losing is what keeps life interesting. If we lose all the time however then we acquire learned helplessness, where we stop trying and we die. We like watching other people lose in life because it makes them human. When we see people's flaws it's re-assuring to us that other people are just like us - human. As I said earlier in the book, a guy's main goal is to sleep with the girl. What happened in this story however was that the main goal was guaranteed: I merely had to follow the recipe. As much as this is attractive (i.e.: it's fail proof), it's actually a turn off as she's totally defeated the most exciting part of a relationship: the chase. The exciting thing about dating and looking for love is the possibility of losing that love at any moment or gaining that love just when you thought things were bleak. The contract

So, Where's My Girlfriend?

she put out in front of me de-humanized the entire courtship process and sometimes, a sure thing is not a good thing.

A Permission to be Porno – One of the most interesting parts of Rosa's proposal was the offer that she would do anything I wanted in the bedroom like it was a favor. The assumption here is that there are things guys want to do with girls in the bedroom that girls will usually not suggest themselves. Guys and girls are not only different in the way they talk and think but also in the way they want to have sex. For example, a common theme I find that guys always want is to have sex with the girl with the lights on. It's because guys are visual creatures and we want to see the whole thing unravel in front of us. One thing that bothers me is when some girls have their eyes closed during sex. I've been told that some girls close their eyes because they think it's weird to be staring at each other during sex. Other girls have flatly told me that they fantasize about somebody else during sex which can't be good for the guy who's currently on top of her. I also think that guys want to do a lot of porno style positions which girls have told me aren't very comfortable. Porno sex is not realistic sex – realistic sex is usually very boring. You have to keep in mind that porno sex is created with the sole intention of performing for the third party (i.e. the guy filming it) Real sex is usually between two people. Who cares if you're not doing porno positions? As long as it feels good, do it. Going back to Rosa's suggestion, she was pretty much allowing me to have uncomfortable sex with her. I can see the novelty of porno sex for a bit but after a while, I'm sure I'll start feeling bad for her and revert back to regular sex. So much for that clause in the contract.

Things you do for Love – I was once told by my female friend that girls don't find getting the money shot sexy at all. I was shocked to hear that female pornstars only pretend to enjoy the money shots which led me to ask her why regular girls do it, if they hated it. Her answer was simple yet enlightening: "I do it because it's sexy." The things people do in order to be sexy ranges widely: I really don't care if I'm fit or fat but in the sake of "being sexy", I reluctantly hit the gym and watch what I eat. No matter what you say, it's still a superficial society we live in. When it comes to sex however there are

So, Where's My Girlfriend?

some unique issues that affect guys and girls. For guys, there's an expectation that he must want sex all the time and that it's unmanly to turn down sex. As unique individuals, we vary in our sex drives where some guys need to constantly have sex (i.e. Eric Benet) while other guys are happy not having a lot of sex (i.e. Online gamers). It's kind of a weird scenario: to find excuses to turn down sex but it's a real issue. Girls on the other hand, are constantly pressured to give in and act like pornstars in bed while maintaining a good girl image outside of the bedroom. Just like my friend says, sometimes girls have to be pornstars in bed because that's what the guy wants and they want the guy to only sleep at her bed and not another girls'. Chris Rock stated it best when he talks about what guys and girls are "accustomed to": once girls are "accustomed" to a certain lifestyle like riding in a nice car, she can never go back to riding the bus. Guys on the other hand, once they're "accustomed" to freaky things in bed, they can never date a girl who won't do the same things his ex did. There's this slippery slope that the girl has to keep matching in order to keep the guy happy. If you want to make your guy stop asking to do kinky stuff, delete all his porn so that he can't get any more ideas.

So, Where's My Girlfriend?

How To Lose A Girl By Treating Her Like A Total Whore

(I wish I could have made up a classier title, but essentially this is what the story is about)

Bill Buckner, Kevin Federline and Me…what do these people have in common? They blew a sure thing.

It's like finding a trunk full of money in my backyard and having it blow away by forgetting to close the trunk. This is what happened to me when I came across a rarity: a girl who was willing to have casual sex. Similar to unicorns, dragons and the yeti, the "fuck friend" is often the object of mythological status since it is often spoken about but almost impossible to verify by the general population. Since the dawn of time, people have always challenged the notion that sex can come without the proverbial strings attached. Whether it's an emotional connection or a bout with syphilis, sex always seems to leave a mark between the parties involved. I'm not referring to a one-time "*I met her at an alley in Mexico*" encounter. I'm talking about multiple encounters with a friend. So, one fine summer, I had a chance to test the age-old question: "*Is it possible to sustain a relationship based purely on sex?*"

 I first met Kendra when I was in high school. She was a year older and she went to a different high school. She was a small girl, perhaps 5'1 and she was cute as hell. She had a boyfriend at that time so she was about as sexy as penicillin to me. You see, I had twisted morals back then – I thought that if a girl was in a relationship, then I shouldn't try and see her in a sexual way. I really took the Bible to heart and tried not to covet my neighbor's wife. Years passed and Kendra and I went our separate ways. I went to university and graduated and she did whatever the hell she did. It's not relevant. Here's the relevant part:

So, one day, I saw her name on a social networking site. One thing I like about technology is the ability for me to keep tabs on people whom I have totally forgotten about. Luckily, at this point, I've already been totally devoid of any moral decency so I began to check her profile out. I looked at Kendra's pictures and I said, "*Wow, this girl is still really cute.*" To add cocaine to my cornflakes, I noticed something about her relationship status: Single.

So, Where's My Girlfriend?

I was determined to raise our relationship back from the dead so I immediately went to work and established contact with her. Before I knew it, we had a date set up. Well, it wasn't a romantic date or anything. I was sneaky and used the excuse of catching up as a guise for a dinner meeting. I call it *The Boiled Frog* method. Apparently, (I don't boil frogs so I wouldn't know) the proper way to boil a frog is to put Kermit in cold water and to gradually turn up the heat. Before poor Kermit notices, he's dinner for Pierre. If you put Kermit straight into boiling water, he would jump off faster than Miss Piggy on an exercise program. So the key word here is: *subtlety.*

The first date was at a nice restaurant. We chatted and ate. We caught up with stuff. We also had wine, which gave me the extra courage I needed to ask her a question (notice the *subtlety* of my probing):

Me: *"So, have you ever had casual sex before?"*
Her: *"Yeah. One time with this guy"*
Me: *"Would you ever do it again...with ME?"* (Again, the key word here is: *"subtlety"*)
Her: *"I would."*

Whoa, what just happened there? No slap? No gasp? No wine on my face? It was so ridiculous that I actually didn't know how to proceed. This never happened to me before so I didn't know how to go about it. We finished our meal and I drove her home. I was happy that I got a verbal agreement from Kendra that she would have casual sex with me. So...now what?

I didn't know how this thing worked. Was there some sort of rulebook? Did Emily Post write about the etiquette on casual sex? I didn't know so I did what a deer in front of headlights would do: I did nothing and hoped that I didn't get injured.

Well, I did something: I took her clubbing the next time and we had fun. At the end of the night, before I dropped her home, I gave her a quick open mouth kiss. She looked surprised by it and quickly went inside. Did I break some rule?

So the next time I met her, I was totally baffled by how this casual sex thing worked. Keeping with the theme of *subtlety,* I asked her:

So, Where's My Girlfriend?

"So, how does this work? Do you want to set up an appointment or something?"

Looking back, I can't believe that she let me get away with so much stupidity. It was either she really wanted me or she was into helping the mentally deficient.

Her reply was: *"We'll just take it naturally and see how things go."*

That might have been fine with her, but for me, I was horny and ready to go. It's like telling your kid that you bought him a kick-ass present for Christmas and when he asks when he can open his gift, you say: *"We'll see"*

I wanted my gift now. I decided that I needed to kick things into action.

For me, putting things into action meant inviting Kendra over to watch some movies. Of course, everyone knows that asking a girl to come over and watch a movie is the codeword for: *"Do you want to come over and fool around?"*

When a girl agrees to come over to watch movies, it's pretty much a green light from the third base coach telling you to make a play for home. I think the defense of *"She agreed to come over and watch movies"* is accepted in court.

She came over and I put in a copy of the television series *The Office*

Two minutes into the show, I put my arm around her.

I know that *The Office* is a funny show and all, but at that point, I didn't care much for it. Sorry Ricky Gervais, I wanted some action.

When I put my arm around her, she pulled away and looked at me.

Then she asked the cursed question: *"Why do you like me?"*

Again, this mole reared its ugly head and I needed to whack it good so that I could get to the buried treasure. I figured that she wanted an answer that I hoped would suffice. Going back to my theme of worst hallmark card answers ever, I managed to pull this out of thin air:

" I think you're really cool and we get along. You're also really funny and have similar interests as me. You make me smile"

So, Where's My Girlfriend?

I guess partly why my answers to this question in these situations are always so horrible is because of the lack of blood in my brain. It's all flowed down to my groin.

I guess her standards for what constituted a good answer was about as high as an entrance exam to a Mexican medical school because my answer was good enough to earn me a make out session with her. So we fooled around but I still wasn't allowed into the castle. I was made to wait outside with my troops.

This standoff didn't last long however as she found herself coming over to watch more movies the very next week. This time, I was sure that she committed to sleeping with me as I fooled around with her while I wore my baseball cap. Who fools around with a guy wearing a hat in bed?

Who knows? Who cares?

So, things got all hot and steamy and before I knew it, she told me to put on the rubber. I did so and soon enough, my army raided the castle and ransacked the place. The villagers were slaughtered and the gold was plundered.

In all honesty, sleeping with Kendra was one of the greatest moments in my life. The pleasure and carnal ecstasy I experienced was beyond this universe. I'm sure that there's a mathematical equation that exists in this universe that can explain the pleasure I felt that night but it's probably never going to be discovered since Satan probably keeps it in a bottle in Hell. If all human beings experienced the pleasure I felt in sleeping with Kendra, there would be no war. Doves will fly all over the world and all we'd do is talk about how ridiculously good we feel all the time. Water cooler talks would consist of the following:

Dave: *"Hey Bill, catch the game last night?"*
Bill: *"Who cares? What about this pleasure we're having????"*
Both in Unison: *"Uhhhhhhhhhhhhhh………"*

Yeah. It was that good.

Observing the law of diminishing returns however, the reason that I speak so highly of my pleasure in sleeping with Kendra was because I was only able to sample the honey one more time before I had it cut off from me, like a vigilant bartender to an alcoholic

So, Where's My Girlfriend?

with the shakes. That's right, I blew it so I wasn't allowed to enter the Promised Land anymore.

So what happened? Well, as human nature dictates, I got cocky and I took things for granted. I assumed that she would come every Sunday like Mass. So the next time we slept together, I quickly rolled off when I finished and got dressed. I told her that I had work the next day and that I was going to drive her home. There was no cuddling or no pillow talk.

I pretty much treated her like a whore.

Looking back, that's probably how she felt.

She didn't raise the issue with me however. She just began to slowly phase me out. She wouldn't reply to my emails, wouldn't pick up my phone calls and soon…she fell off the face of the Earth. A few months after, I ran into her at a birthday party of a shared acquaintance. There she was, with her new boyfriend. She couldn't look at me in the eye. Her boyfriend was also a bit standoffish but I heard that he was an asshole, so fuck him. Perhaps she told him of our little tryst?

No guy likes meeting the guy who slept with his girl.

Whatever.

He can only have their future since I'll always have her past.

Lessons Learned

Smash and Grab – One time, I went to a casino to gamble. I approached the roulette table and proceeded to bet on the colors on the table: Red or Black. I started the game with $50 and within a few minutes, I left the table with $250. Being a novice gambler, it was safe to say that I was fucking ecstatic about winning $200 from the casino. That night, I really felt that I was getting something from nothing.

To feel like you're getting something from nothing is one of the best feelings to experience in life. This is why everyone's obsessed with winning the lottery: it's getting something (i.e. millions of dollars) from virtually nothing ($1 or $2).

So, Where's My Girlfriend?

Transporting this concept to the relationship universe, the feeling of getting something from nothing is best experienced when two people have sex with no-strings attached. Well, specifically guys feel particularly good.

This is the reason why:

There's a biological theory that says that guys and girls are programmed to approach sex very differently from each other. For a guy, the big picture is to make sure his genes are passed down to the next generation therefore the goal is to impregnate as much girls as possible in order to increase the number of off-springs he has. For girls however, the objective is the complete opposite: to have as minimal lovers as possible. The reason being is that the process of childbirth for women is long, painful and dangerous. As a result, women are more selective in choosing a mate since the wrong choice can leave them single mothers. This theory argues that all of these behaviours are derived from our caveman days which made sense: back then, there were no caveman welfare programs or caveman daycares to watch over the kids so if you're a caveman, the best way to increase your odds of genetic survival is to simply play the numbers: have as much kids as possible and hope that some of them make it to a ripe old age of 24.

Fast forward to today's society: despite the absence of saber-tooth tigers threatening our lives, men and women are still on the opposite ends of the spectrum when it comes to sex with men trying to sleep with as much women as possible and women keeping their counts as low as possible (note: does not apply to pornstars). So why is this?

The theory states that it wasn't that long ago when we were cave people. Some habits are just hard to break: just as how we're still naturally averse to snakes, water, etc. (things that used to kill us in the past), we've ingrained this attitude towards sex in our head. Women want the guy to stay around if she gets pregnant to help her raise the child.

As a result, you have guys today trying to get something out of nothing: to have sex with a girl without the monogamous commitment and the financial support that usually accompanies it. Girls on the other hand have put up a series of checklists before she gives up her royal goodies to make sure this doesn't happen. She won't sleep with a guy if she doesn't trust him. If she can't even feel secure giving her credit card number to him, then she probably won't be sleeping with him as well.

So, Where's My Girlfriend?

So what you have is a game of cops and robbers: guys are always out to pull a fast one and sleep with as many girls as possible while the girls are looking to safe proof themselves from these guys by trying to put up bullshit detectors. The funny thing however is that most guys are robbers during their youth: while they have time and don't think about the future. Give them time however and they eventually want to get caught and tied down by a girl…that's when they realize that crime really doesn't pay.

Coming and Going – Here I am talking about how I lost this girl, how I blew a sure thing. In hindsight, maybe I was used by her to get over an ex-boyfriend (or a current boyfriend). I get philosophical about life and destiny and I think that people come and go in your life. Nothing personal – you have friends you grew up with and they leave your life. 20 years later, they come back in your life. Similar to this, there are going to be romantic interests that will come and go in your life. I've known people who were in love but somehow ended up marrying other people and now that they're both divorced, they finally end up together. It's hard not to believe in destiny when stuff like that happens. At the same time, there are some people that are only supposed to play a small role in your life – this can be the person you always see on the subway or the person you slept with three times and never came back. When you mess up a relationship, you have no choice but to be philosophical about it since nothing good comes out of regret. Regrets kill you because you'd always find yourself saying, "*I should have done this instead of that.*" When a relationship fucks up, you can't do anything about it because you can't predict people's behaviours. People are not like tuna casseroles where you can say "I should have added more tuna." So it didn't work out between me and Kendra – we had our fun then she went her separate ways. I try not to think about it but sometimes I do think what would happen had I stayed with her…I guess it's hard being human.

Chemistry 101 – I have some friends that are great to party with but are horrible travel companions. I've gone out with girls that made great arm candy but horrible conversationalists. It's not that there's anything wrong with them; it's an issue of chemistry: perhaps these guys travel well with other people with their travel habits and these girls get along just great with guys on their wavelength. Sometimes, you meet

So, Where's My Girlfriend?

someone that you might not really mesh well with…outside of the bedroom but inside the bedroom is a different story. Finding someone that has great sexual chemistry with you is like finding an honest mechanic: you hold onto that motherfucker because you might not find another one in your lifetime. Then again, it's hard to hold onto someone if the sexual chemistry is the only thing keeping you two together. In the short term, it might work: you're both single and while you date other people, you're still having great sex together. As time marches on however, someone tends to wake up and want out of the conspiracy: either she has found someone she connects with or she wants more than a sexual relationship with you. You're kind of screwed both ways: A) If she found someone she can connect with on a deeper level than you can with her, then she's probably willing to downgrade her sex life to "Mediocre" in return for a more fulfilling dating life with the new guy. B) If she wants a relationship beyond sex with you, we already established earlier that the only chemistry you seem to have with her is in the bedroom. You can try to get to know her better but again, it's hard to force yourself to click with someone. Again, that's the whole point of "chemistry", you can't fake it.

So, Where's My Girlfriend?

The Dreaded Friendzone

Now, I want to talk to you about something that I've yet to figure out. This has eluded me throughout my life and remains one of the greatest unsolved mysteries plaguing Mankind. This mystery has puzzled the Incas, the Greek philosophers and made John Hinckley Jr. shoot President Regan. This is the mystery of the *Friendzone*.

There was this girl I really liked once. She was cute, witty and very cool. I wanted to date her and live happily ever after with her. Of course, that didn't happen since I missed my chance. Some opportunities in life happen only once: Rookie of the Year, getting selected first overall in the NBA draft and getting a power boost in Super Mario Kart. When it comes to girls, guys only have a small window of opportunity to sell themselves as a potential mate before they either:

1) Get rejected
2) Get accepted
3) Get put in the *Friendzone*.

Ask any guy; once a girl thinks he's "*only a friend*", it's rare to ever transition from being friends to becoming lovers. I believe that it's probably better to be outright rejected by the girl and to never see her again than to endure the constant pain of being in her *Friendzone*. For the uneducated, here's a brief summary of what it means to be in the *Friendzone*:

Boy likes girl but girl is not sure about dating boy so she innocently suggests, *"Why don't we be friends instead?"* Boy agrees to this, hoping in his poor little heart that he can win her over romantically by being a great friend. Little does boy know that he's just been officially placed in the *Friendzone*. Once boy is in that zone, he will never see the inside of her pants because the *Friendzone* is a black hole. The reason is that boy can't win her romantically anymore as girl no longer thinks of boy in a romantic way. To girls, friends and lovers are as distinct as night and day.

So, Where's My Girlfriend?

When a guy becomes a "friend" to a girl he really wants to date, it means that he settled. For some reason, he couldn't win her romantically so he took the plea bargain and decided to be a friend to her instead. This is a bad choice since this is the same feeling of Prometheus getting pecked by birds for the rest of his immortal life: the guy would have to endure constant pain over a long period of time. Being put in the *Friendzone* hurts because most guys never wanted friendship in the first place but somehow, they ended up there.

To reiterate, a guy settled and is now reminded of that sting every time he sees this girl. Oh, she'll hug and kiss him alright…but only as a friend. Many guys have made this mistake and many more will make this mistake. This seems to be some sort of Rite of Passage that every guy in the world seems to need to experience at least one time in his life. I think what makes this concept of *Friendzone* especially bothersome for a guy is that he always thinks that the girl should always be dating better quality guys than the ones she's currently dating. Specifically, she should be dating…him.

Here is an example: Boy likes girl but is hesitant to make a move. Now it's too late and girl has placed boy in the *Friendzone*. Reluctantly, boy accepts his lot in her life just because he is still obsessed with her. Now that the two are "good buddies", girl proceeds to tell boy about every creepy guy and asshole she dates (after all, this is what good friends do – they share dating stories). Girl rubs salt on boy's wounds when she tells him about how guys sleep with her but stop calling her shortly after. Guy automatically gets upset upon hearing this but doesn't know why.

Here are the two reasons why: First, boy is upset because he can't seem to understand how blind this girl is – there's a perfectly good guy (i.e.: him) who would treat her like a princess but she just can't see it. Instead, she prefers to get jerked around by asshole guys. Secondly, boy is upset because he can't believe that this asshole got away with sleeping with her (which is what he really wanted to do) without doing all the boyfriend duties. Actually, it seems like boy is the one doing all the duties while the guys she dates get a free ride. That's the thing about being in Friendzone – its boyfriend duties without boyfriend benefits.

So, Where's My Girlfriend?

So I met Carla through a mutual friend during the time I was going out with my girlfriend in university. When a guy meets girls while he's already in a relationship, these girls automatically put him in the *Friendzone* because usually, girls are mindful of taking the boyfriend of other girls.

Years passed by and I somehow kept in touch with Carla. There were times when she was single and there were times when I was single until finally, we hit a point when we were both single. As friends, we spent a lot of time going out. We started doing couply things like going to dinners and going to parties together. Soon, I really wanted to be more than a friend to Carla.

Cue Usher's song "*You Make Me Wanna*"

Before anything came between us
You were like my bestfriend
The one I used to run to when me and my
Girl was having problems
You used to say it would be okay
Suggest little nice things I should do
And when I come home at night and lay my head down
All I seem to think about is you
And how you make me wanna

(Chorus)
You make me wanna leave the one I'm with
Start a new relationship with you
This is what you do
Think about her and the things that come along with
You make me
You make me wanna leave the one I'm with
Start a new realtionship with you

So, Where's My Girlfriend?

I kept disclosing my feelings about Carla to my close friends until one day, my friend
says, *"You should just tell her how you feel and see what happens"*
In other words:

Fuck it.

"Fuck it", said Christopher Columbus when he found out he was going the wrong way.
"Fuck it", said Albert Einstein when he wasn't sure if E did equal MC squared
"Fuck it", said Mark, when he contemplated telling Carla how he felt about her.

Plenty of times, I made subtle suggestions to Carla about how good we looked as a
couple or how well we got along. One time, I suggested that she was my weekend
girlfriend. Finally, I decided to blow the whistle and call it like I see it.
So on one occasion, I suggested to her that we should date because we were compatible
and so good for each other. This is what she said to me:

*"I don't have a lot of close guy friends. I think what we have here is special and I don't
want to blow it. I have a habit of breaking up with guys for my own stupid reasons and I
don't want to lose our friendship"*

At first, I was sold. Then I began to ask my other girlfriends about what she said. They
all told me that it was a line. Apparently, if a girl really liked you, she would risk her
friendship to go out with you.
In other words, she would have said, *"Fuck it."*
This made me sad and upset.
One day, I saw Carla online so I messaged her and brought up the idea of going out
again. Just like before, she blew me off with a generic line. This led me to suggest to her
that our relationship was like the irony that was constant in the relationship between Lois
Lane and Clark Kent. For me, it was like I could never go out with Carla or else it would
be too perfect – I would actually be happy and life wouldn't seem so painful. Alas, that's

So, Where's My Girlfriend?

not possible as experiencing a brief moment of happiness doesn't seem to fit in with the tragedy that is my life. Perhaps in my next life would I be as happy as a clam.

After I mentioned this observation, Carla enquired "*So, I'm Lois Lane?*"

I replied: "*Yes, and if you really knew who I was, I'd pleasantly surprise you*" (I didn't want to say something like "*You would find out that I'm Superman*" since it felt like a sexual innuendo that associated me with having an overly large manhood or coming faster than a speeding bullet)

With that response, she again referred to the need to keep things where they were. As a friend, she found me incredible and mind-blowing. I guess that in today's world, those qualities don't necessarily translate to the make-up of a good boyfriend.

I told her that she was being near-sighted and that she was being irrational. This is when I knew that I was in trouble: I had to rationalize and convince a girl to go out with me. In fact, I dug deeper and said this about our relationship:

"We're like a foreign song you hear on the radio. You like it a lot but you don't know what the singer is saying so you put your own ideas and feelings into it. At the end, you never want to know what they're really saying because it would never compare to your own interpretation of it. We put our hopes and ideals into the other person because we know that as long as we never truly get to know them, they'll never disappoint us."

After that, she quickly logged off which suggested that she didn't like what I had to say. The bottom line is that even Superman and foreign songs can't get me out of the *Friendzone.*

So, Where's My Girlfriend?

Lessons Learned

"It's very expensive" – There was a scene in "Pretty Woman" when Julia Roberts enters a high-end clothing store looking to buy some clothes that were the opposite of "Hookerish". When she enquired about the price of a certain dress, the snobby saleslady replied in a coded manner, "*It's very expensive.*" At first, she didn't get it so she asked the saleswoman again. She got the same reply, "*It's very expensive.*" With that, Julia Roberts got the message and ran out of the store crying her hooker eyes out.

Sometimes, the friends we fall in love with act like the snobby saleswoman when we tell them how we've fallen in love with them. They might say, "*That's probably not a good idea.*" or "*You're just confused.*" I think underneath their coded replies, they mean well and don't want to hurt us. What they're trying to say is this:

"It's quite evident that you've fallen in love with me. I've taken this possibility into consideration by performing counterfactual thought experiments in my head but have decided that it's probably not in our best interest to pursue this particular course of action. However, I do treasure your friendship and your generosity to drive me to see my dentist during my days off therefore I would like to keep our friendship. I will save you the embarrassment of flatly rejecting you by giving you a coded message and I shall pray to God that you get the hint. Perhaps you're not as stupid as you look."

Guys, be aware that girls give these coded messages all the time. Girls are very subtle in the way they get their message across. Here is a sample of coded messages I have gotten throughout my years of humiliation and rejection:

"I love you so much as a friend and I cherish our friendship. I don't want to ruin it by taking a chance at a relationship."

"I need to take some time to think about this." (This is not okay if she gives you this reply for three years in a row now)

"I see you more as a big brother. You're almost like family to me."

So, Where's My Girlfriend?

How you know it's a coded message for rejection:

If you're not sure what a girl means by her answer, the solution is to find a trusted girl friend and ask her for her opinion. The key to understanding girl language is to recruit a girl to work for you – how simple is that?

So I have a team of girls who are at my beck and call ready to translate girl talk to me. This is what I learned from them: If a girl likes you enough, she'd be willing to risk her friendship with you in order to be with you romantically. In other words, using the excuse of "not ruining the friendship" is utter bullshit. A girl will act on her feelings first then rationalize them later to fit the situation. For guys on the other hand…sometimes, we need to have it spelt out for us.

Guys and Friendzone

Had Julia Roberts been a guy in "Pretty Woman", this would have been the dialogue that took place:

Male Julia: *"How much is this dress?"*

Snobby shopkeeper: *"It's very expensive."*

Male Julia: *"What do you mean?"*

Snobby shopkeeper: *"It's very expensive."*

Male Julia: *"But I want to buy it. What do you mean?"*

Snobby shopkeeper: *"You're a hooker and we don't think you have enough STD laced money to buy our high-end stuff. We're trying to get you out of our store before other people see you."*

Male Julia: *"Oh, I see. So I can't buy this?"*

What this means is that when guys confront girls about being more than friends, they usually get their hearts broken because they're too stupid to get the hint. At this point, the girl would have to list reasons as to why they can't go out. Usually, she doesn't list the one that hurts the most: she just doesn't have feelings for him. Being an idiot, guys will usually fight to convince the girl that they should be going out and have rebuttals for each reason she has given. If he ever finds himself at this stage of the argument, he would be wise to realize that he's already lost if he has to appeal to rationality and logical thinking

So, Where's My Girlfriend?

in order to win the girl's heart. It's pretty tough to convince a girl to like you by out-arguing her. What kind of response would a guy expect?

"Fine! You win! I'll like you!"

Maybe there is a way to win a girl's heart through rationality. The secret exists but there's a price for it. You want to know the price?

It's very expensive.

Love Re-examined – I think that falling in love with a friend is a very common occurrence. To understand this issue better, we need to talk about what friendship is and how it differs from romance. It is my opinion that the line separating friends from lovers is a thin white chalk, which blows according to the wind. Some people become friends before they fall in love and get married while other people get married, get divorced and end up becoming friends. One thing in common in friendship and romance is this: you like the other person but to what extent?

Some people love their friends more than they love their spouses. I think we're seeing this all wrong: we tend to assume that there's only one type of love and the only thing we can do is vary the intensity of this love according to our relationship with people. For example, the love intensity for acquaintances is 2/10. For friends, it's 6/10. For family, it's 8/10 and for your partner, 9/10.

Given our the complexities in Life, I tend to side more with the Greek thinking that there are different types of love in this world from *eros* to *agape*. Here's a really random example:

If you're hunting animals in a safari, using one type of gun probably isn't enough to hunt all the animals in the wild. You may be able to use your revolver to kill that prairie dog but you'll probably need a rifle to hunt that lion and that elephant gun to shoot Dumbo. So similar to Love, you can hunt all kinds of animals with only one type of weapon, but that would be kind of stupid and you'll probably get killed by an elephant.

On Second Thought – I think falling in love with a friend is similar to going to a buffet: at first it sounds like a good idea but at the end of your meal, you might be re-thinking your decision. A lot of people don't think through their decisions when it comes to

So, Where's My Girlfriend?

romancing their friends. One might think that there are only upsides to this: you both already know each other well, your parents know her parents and you already share the same group of friends. So, what could possibly change the relationship?

Sex.

To explain this better, we need to rewind all the way to the beginning of your friendship and how it started. **This is the first insight about guys: guys are always looking for sex.** Chris Rock is right on the ball when he talks about guys and offering dick: everything a guy does for a girl, he's offering his dick. When guys are nice to a girl, it's because he wants to sleep with her. This is true just as the skies are blue. So, what about friendship between guys and girls? Again, quoting Chris Rock: friendship is where a guy ends up when he screws up and instead of sleeping with her, ends up in friendzone.

So now, you have a situation where most guys are reluctantly friends with girls. It was never their intention but they somehow got marooned on this lonely island. Now, they have to settle for an arrangement where they have to hear the girl's sex stories about douchebag guys and how guys just sleep with her and then never call. It pains the male friend to hear this stuff as they could have easily been that guy who's now avoiding her phone calls. Instead, they've been relegated to human pillows where she rests her head and waits for the next douchebag to physically and mentally ruin her.

You might be thinking: why doesn't the guy just leave the friendship if it pains him so much? **Here is the second insight about guys: guys never give up when it comes to trying to get sex.** Sure she's treating him like a eunuch but if the girl is hot enough, a guy will hang on and keep chipping away at her, hoping that one day she capitulates to his perverted fantasy. A guy might tell a girl that he loves her like a sister, but in the back of his mind, he's ready to love her like a half sister. So comes the rationale about dating a friend: if we get along, then why don't we just go out and have sex with each other? Hence, the question all guys must ask themselves before they go and start falling in love with their female friends is this:

Do I really love her or do I just want to sleep with her?

A lot of times, guys think they love someone but in the end, they realize that they just want to sleep with a girl. So, how can one not get tripped up?

The answer is this: **Always see her at her worst.**

So, Where's My Girlfriend?

That's right: make an effort to see her only when she's not wearing makeup and is wearing her mom's flannel pajamas. Try and hang out with her when she just finished spin classes and smells like ass. That is the ultimate test: if you still want to be with this girl despite all these ungodly distractions, then it might be the time to jump on it.

So, Where's My Girlfriend?

My Black Swan

This story is one of those that I still can't get over to this day. Whenever I look back, I can't believe it happened. Like a perfect game in bowling or the perfect steak, you sort of get sad that you might never experience such bliss again.

This is my story:

It was the week of a film festival and my friend wanted me to check out a movie with her. Since she worked in media, she got us access to all the movies and the after parties that followed. On a crisp Wednesday night, I met up with her to take in a movie. The movie kinda sucked but what was important was the after party. Since my friend had an early morning the next day, she declined in joining me in attending the after party, which was being held at a nearby club. So after the movie finished, she left and I was alone. Never the one to be deterred from partying on a weeknight, I called up my friend Ken.

Similar to me, Ken never turns down an opportunity to have a good time. We entered the club only to find it kind of empty. Again, being a weeknight, many of the moviegoers opted to go home. What we had left were people that were either: the organizers, people in the industry, people trying to get into the industry and unemployed party boys like me. Upon entering the club, a cute, petite, long-haired Asian girl walked by with her friend. I quickly concluded that this girl was the most attractive girl in the room so my targets were set directly at her. I wanted to get her attention but I didn't have anything to say. I did notice that she was eating hors d'oeuvres, which gave me the reason to strike up a conversation:

Me: *"Excuse me, where did you get that?"*
Her: *"Over there, it's pretty good."*
Me: *"I can see that from the way you're eating it with no shame."*
Her: *"I'm hungry and I don't care that I'm eating in front of people."*
Me: *"Blah...blah...blah"*

So, Where's My Girlfriend?

Eventually, I learned some valuable information about the two girls. They were friends and they were in town for the film festival. The Asian girl, Kim, was an aspiring actress and writer. Her friend Reena, was the director. So they kind of had a Matt Damon/Ben Affleck thing going on. As well, they were from out of town and were only planning on staying for the weekend.

As the night progressed, I continued talking to Kim. I asked her questions about acting and her project. She was glad to oblige me with answers and I kept learning more things about her. At this point, I contemplated about asking her for her number but at the same time, I have a bad habit of not asking for a girl's number until it's too late. It's kind of weird to ask a girl for her number right off the bat since I haven't had the time to really get to know her. My girl friends seem to agree with this. It's just weird to say,

"Hi, I'm blah blah blah. What's your name? Wow, that's such a unique name…so can I get your number?"

This is a big problem for me since I always hesitate to pull the number trigger until it's too late. Usually I see the girl at the beginning of the evening and I assume that I'll probably run into her again. Unfortunately, I usually don't see her again for the rest of the night. At the same time, I find that I've been relying on the excuse *"it's too early to get her number"* so much that it really has become my excuse to wimp out in asking for a number. I wonder when it's actually the right time to ask for a number? I'm guessing there's no universal "after 15 minutes" rule (although it would be funny if there was a universal 15 minute rule and you could buy a clock that would ring once fifteen minutes is up: RIIIINGGG!!! … "So, can I have your number?")

I know the answer is probably something wishy washy like: *"It's probably something that depends on the level of connection you're making with the girl."*

I don't like that answer because it leaves too much room for miscommunication. Girls have told me repeatedly about moments when they've waited impatiently for the guy to ask for their number. The fruit is ripe for the picking but most guys don't pick it since most guys don't know how to tell when a fruit is ripe. Girls, next time just help a guy out and say, *"So, do you want my number?"*

So, Where's My Girlfriend?

I suggested to Kim that we should hang out the next time she was in town. She did me one better: *"Why don't I give you my number?"*
I guess she took my suggestion.
So she proceeded to give me her business card and contact number. After chatting for several more minutes, her and her friend called it a night and went home. The next day, I added her on my Facebook and we started a conversation. Maintaining a good Facebook site is very important as Facebook is all about personal branding. This is where you are able to influence what other people will think of you when they check out your profile. For me, my profile consisted of a lot of party photos. This is to relay the message to other people that I have a social life and girls don't find me creepy. If a profile consists of photos of a guy in his basement displaying his assortment of guns and hunting knives, that might give off the creepy vibe just a bit.

Apparently, Kim was the type of girl that did her homework. She had already scoped out my Facebook page and I had checked out. She considered me friendly, sociable and trustworthy. We proceeded to have a chat online for several hours just to learn more about each other. I guess it was an online date or a pre-assessment for a possible date. Kim and I hit it off as she called me the next day and we agreed to go watch a movie.
I got to the movie theatre early so I decided to walk around the street to think. I was puzzled as to the reason why she was hanging out with me. Was this a friendship thing or a romantic thing? Is this a date or just hanging out? The thought of her using me entered my mind. It's like if I were on vacation, it would be nice to have a local show me around. Eventually, Kim arrived and we met before the movie started. As we waited in line, I asked where her best friend Reena was. Kim told me that Reena was at another event but she was going to drop by later on.
Oh man. Talk about a cockblock.
Eventually, Reena came by and began to chat with us. I was afraid she would join us thereby becoming a buffer zone between Kim and me so I innocently inquired:
"So Reena, will you be joining us?" (Emphasis on the word "us")
She replied: *"No, I don't think so. I'm pretty tired."*
With that, she bid us adieu and left.

So, Where's My Girlfriend?

Finally, the doors of the movie theatre opened and we proceeded inside.
Soon after, the movie ended. I asked her where she wanted to go next and she told me
that she'd been craving some Vietnamese food. With that, I whisked her away to
Chinatown where we found a restaurant that satisfied her craving. The meal consisted of
some good conversation about light topics like family and career. Soon, the conversation
switched to the holy trinity of taboo: sex, religion and politics. Thankfully, we seemed to
share similar views on all three, especially sex. She was pretty cool with sex and she
thought that girls shouldn't have to be ashamed of sleeping with a guy. We talked about
the differences in perspective between guys and girls and I told her that as a guy, I would
never refuse a girl if she wanted to sleep with me. At this point, she asked me what I
usually did to take a girl home. I told her that one time, I forgot something back at my
place so I had to take the girl back to my house. Upon reaching my place, I asked the girl
if she wanted to see my room. The girl says yes, and we'll just say we didn't make it to
the movies.
After dinner was over, it was getting late and she needed to be up bright and early the
next day. I would have considered the night a success already if she asked me to take her
straight home. I asked her where she wanted me to take her next,
She said: *"How about you show me your room?"*

It's hard to hold in a smile after a girl has just pretty much told you that she wants to go
back to your place. I'm sure Alex Rodriguez felt the same way when the New York
Yankees gave him a $100 million contract. So, she wanted to see my room, I gladly
obliged and got her into my car. During the car ride, I felt nervous. I was given the ball
and all I had to do was not drop it. The last thing I wanted to do was say the wrong thing
that would have her getting out of the car so I played the car ride home really cool. If you
want to play it cool, just don't say anything. Just shut the hell up.

Soon enough, we arrived at my house. At first, I played the humble host: asking her if she
wanted something to drink and stuff like that. I also gave her the short tour of my room.
Soon, it dawned on me: How is this supposed to work? Should I start stripping? Do I
have to sweet talk her? Again, I never received the email regarding the protocols of such

procedures. Suddenly, all the memories of my previous experiences of casual sex with girls (please refer back to "How To Lose A Girl By Treating Her Like A Whore") came flooding back.

First, I excused myself and went to the washroom to freshen up. This meant a quick brush of my teeth so I wouldn't smell like an extra from *Lord of The Rings*. As well, I made a quick examination of how I looked. In a tribute to John Travolta ala *Saturday Night Fever*, I made sure my hair was set perfectly. After I finished, she asked to use the washroom as well which gave me time to think of my next step. While she was in the washroom, I wasn't sure what I was supposed to be doing.

Should I be sitting, waiting patiently like a kid waiting for his parents after soccer practice? Should I be pretending to read an encyclopedia in my underwear, acting like she interrupted my thirst to know about Ancient Greece?

I decided to play it safe and turn off all the lights except a small lamp beside my bed. I also decided to jump into bed and wait for her. I think this was a good option as opposed to standing outside the door waiting for her, naked except for my socks.

When she came out, she saw me in bed waiting for her. I didn't know how she was going to react. Well, she reacted pretty well as she proceeded to literally jump on top of me and straddle me. What's with girls and straddling?

So we slept together and afterwards, during pillow talk, I found out that Kim had recently broke up with her boyfriend and she just needed some tender loving care. I loved her reasoning: *"Just because I'm single doesn't mean that I can't enjoy sex."*

Very true my dear.

I also inquired about her friend Reena.

I asked Kim whether Reena knew what she was up to tonight. Kim's response surprised me: *"It was actually Reena's idea that I do this."*

So, it appears that the cockblock turned out to be a cockfriend. I felt bad for doubting Reena after. She's like that guy in the first Harry Potter movie that turned out to be a good guy. Then came the big part: I was also hesitant to bring up "the talk" – I didn't know what sleeping with her meant: Was I now in a relationship? Did she expect me to start calling? Again, what's the protocol? I decided to stick to a very simple plan: just shut up and don't bring it up. It was my understanding that this was a casual thing and I hoped that Kim felt the same way. Fortunately, Kim also saw this as a casual thing. Eventually, it got late and I drove her back to her hotel. Upon reaching her hotel, I turn to her to say goodbye. At this point, I was expecting a sentimental goodbye.

She turns to me and says: *"Well, thanks for a good time. Bye!"* and proceeds to slam the door.

Lessons Learned

Saying a lot by saying nothing – When I was in highschool, I quickly learned a rule to obey in order to stay out of trouble: shut the hell up.

Even if I know who threw the protractor that nailed the teacher in the head, I would obey the rule of keeping quiet. I know it's cowardly but I did it for my own physical and social self-preservation: the level of justice my teacher sought in finding the perpetrator was unequal to the level of pain I was probably going to experience after class if I were to snitch on my classmate. I have to see these people for four years of my life.

This concept of keeping your mouth shut extends outside the high school code. In prison, people who snitch are usually stabbed in the yard with a fork. Even in the court system, it is within every American's right not to answer questions. In other words, it is our natural right to shut the hell up.

Keeping quiet also comes in very handy in relationships and dating, especially when you're not sure about the status between you and your lover. For example, you're seeing this person but at the same time, you're also talking to a few potential candidates. If nobody brings up the topic of "being exclusive", then the default assumption is that you are free to date other people. Usually, the person who realizes that he's dating way above his league would be keen to have "the talk" with his partner in an effort to lock her in, like a fixed mortgage rate. For the girl who's still shopping around for better guys, she might be reluctant to have that talk. In fact, she won't bring it up until she absolutely has to.

So it makes common sense – people who think they're getting a good deal out of the relationship are always the ones who are keen to have the talk. What happens when both

So, Where's My Girlfriend?

people think that they can do better than the current people they're seeing and don't want to commit to anything?

They both shut the hell up.

 That's the beauty of silence – it gives people an excuse to do things they "assumed" were okay: *"But honey, since nothing was said, I assumed that it was okay to sleep with your sister!"*

At the same time, keeping silent is the option people take when they don't want to be the one tasked to define the relationship. Usually when someone says *"Can we talk about us?"* this means that she can no longer take this game of ambiguity and needs to know the rules and boundaries that come with the relationship. She has just brought the relationship out to light and will now have to be defined as either a monogamous relationship, a booty call or friendship, etc.

Remember, if it looks like a duck, sounds like a duck and walks like a duck, it's not a duck until someone says it is.

Roman Holiday – To know something about someone's ethics, ask her the following question:

Imagine that there are ten people in front of you. Amongst that ten, nine are murderers while one is completely innocent. There is NO WAY to find out who the innocent person is.

Now, would you either:

1. Free them all?
   OR
2. Send them all to prison?

The way the person answers reflects their ethics: if she chooses to free them all, then she believes in a Deontological approach. You're probably wondering what that means. Well, here it is according to Wikipedia:

...Deontologists look at rule and duties. For example, the act may be considered the right thing to do even if it produces a bad consequence ...

So, Where's My Girlfriend?

In this case, the right thing to do is to let everyone go since it is wrong to punish innocent people. The bad consequence is that nine murderers go free. The justice system in most Western countries reflect this rationale which is why everyone is assumed to be innocent until they are found guilty beyond a reasonable doubt. I can't say the same about North Korea.

Oppositely, if you go with the option of sending everyone to prison, then you're more of a Utilitarian. Again, Wikipedia says:

...Utilitarianism is often described by the phrase "the greatest good for the greatest number of people", and is also known as "the greatest happiness principle".

In this case, the greatest good is to take nine murders off the streets thereby protecting the lives of thousands of other people. The negative impact of one innocent person suffering in jail is not equivalent to the safety of thousands. Sorry dude.

So asking this question tells you a lot about someone's ethics. You can also ask a similar question to find out someone's dating ethics, specifically what their ethics are in regards to sleeping with people who are usually below their standards.

Normally, people don't sleep with people below their standards. That's the whole point of having standards. In some cases however, this standard is perverted or straight out ignored. Specifically, standards go down the drain when people find themselves on vacation. So here is the ethical question:

Imagine that you're on vacation at a resort. Being single, you're looking for some romance on your trip however there's one problem: everyone at the resort is super ugly. As your vacation slowly comes to an end, you finally get accosted by a super ugly patron who wants to sleep with you. The rationale is this:

We're both on vacation and no one will ever know.

You think about it for a while and realize that this person is right – he lives halfway across the world and you will probably never see this person again. In fact, you don't

So, Where's My Girlfriend?

even know his name and vice versa. I guess the only thing stopping you is his super ugliness.

So, you have only two choices:

1. Not sleep with this person

   OR

2. Sleep with this person

First, let's talk about not sleeping with this person and the insights we can derive from this. If you don't sleep with this person, it probably means that you have a good understanding of yourself and your values. You probably know yourself well enough to foresee the guilt or remorse that would probably accompany you after the trip if you were to sleep with this person. As well, you have your standards and you don't compromise on them even if you're on vacation. You have a rule: I don't sleep with ugly people no matter where I am. Then again, it is also possible that you're a risk-adverse person and that you don't like to do wild and crazy things like sleeping with a random ugly stranger who's potentially swimming with sexually transmitted diseases. Perhaps this is a good thing since you might bring back more than a suntan from your vacation.

If you did sleep with this person, it might say something about you. First of all, it might mean that you're a risk taker or a fun loving person. Hey, when you're on vacation…then anything goes right? I think we've all known someone who's done something like this. I confess that I have had some regrettable adventures during my past vacations.

That's the insight I wanted to talk about – when some people are on vacation, anything goes…including their values and standards.

Going on vacation is a funny thing: people do crazy stuff they would normally never do in their home town. It could be due to a bevy of reasons: in a foreign country, nobody knows who you are and will probably never see you again so you don't really care what people think of you. On the same circumstance, you can role play and be a somebody since you're a nobody in your home country – just ask English teachers in Japan. Whatever the reason is, one thing is apparent – people's values and standards seem to get left on the airport check-in counter so what does this all mean?

Tourists are easy.

So, Where's My Girlfriend?

If you meet a tourist in your hometown, there's probably a good chance that you might be able to sleep with him mainly from the fact that he's a tourist and he forgot his values at the airport counter. Now, does this mean that you're below his regular standards? Maybe.

At the same time, you can see it the other way: he's a tourist and you'll probably never see him again so you don't mind going below YOUR standards to sleep with him. At least it gives him a good memory of visiting your country which is way better than a shitty postcard.

For guys who meet female tourists, one big thing working for them is the short time window tourists have. Unless they plan to stay for a month, most tourists usually visit a city for a few days or a week. What this means is that first dates automatically become second dates and so on. For example, the furthest you might be able to go with a local girl on a first date is usually a hug (or a kiss on the cheek if you're lucky). On second dates, the best case scenario is usually a kiss. On tourist dating time however I think that it's acceptable to already be on kissing terms on the first date. You're having sex in her hotel room on the second date. It's dating on speed.

How to get laid easily

There's an urban legend about a quote from the famous bank robber, Willie Sutton. When asked why he robbed banks, Sutton was reported as saying,

"Because that's where the money is"

Applying this simple rationale into the world of tourist fucking, if you're looking to meet tourists, it would probably be in your best interest to hang out in tourist-rich areas. Every major city in North America usually has tourist "hot spots" (aka places tourists think are "local" but are actually tourist traps) where tourists congregate. Just hang out there and I'm sure you'll meet a lot of tourists. Alternatively, you can think big and go to locations where there are only tourists: resorts and Las Vegas. Going to these places will definitely increase your chances of scoring as these places are essentially meeting places for tourists to hook up (Note: this would probably not apply to Disney Resorts). The lesson here is ironic: the next time you want to sleep with a tourist, leave your country.

So, Where's My Girlfriend?

Dating 2.0 and the wonders of Technology – Before the Internet, it was pretty difficult for people to get access to sex. If you lived in a farm in the middle of bum-fuck nowhere your choices for getting sex is usually a toss-up between Betsy the Cow versus your curious cousin. With the advent of the Internet however access to sex has never been easier. On one hand, there are very direct sources to access sex: XXX chatrooms, adult websites and dating sites seem to be the basic sources. For the cunning pervert however there are indirect sources for sex: Facebook – let me explain.

Recall earlier in the story that Kim did her due diligence on me by investigating my Facebook page. This is what is called "Facebook creeping". Given Facebook's popularity and the propensity of people to not give a fuck about privacy, it is very easy in today's world to find out a lot of useful information about another person simply by Facebook creeping. There are two main reasons why people Facebook creep: Aside from the obvious desire to learn more about the other person, for guys, they Facebook creep to see if the girl has any hot friends they can hook their chronically single buddies with. For girls, they generally Facebook creep for the purpose of making sure that the guy isn't a serial killer.

So you want to Facebook creep. Aside from what a person writes on his information section, there are also subtle ways to know more about someone on Facebook:

1. **Friends** – having the "Friends in common" feature is very handy as this gives you a context as to who this person might be. Again, if birds of a feather do flock together then it might say something about the person you're Facebook creeping if he has in common all the friends you know that are into Goth. This would probably explain his makeup and his black leather underwear.

2. **Pictures (What you see)** – Pictures are KEY to finding out about someone's character. If the person has pictures of him kayaking, mountain climbing and tree top trekking then I'm willing to bet that he's probably a nature lover. If he has pictures of his gun collection, his collection of stuffed squirrels and his face superimposed on Mount Rushmore then you might want to call the FBI.

3. **Pictures (What you don't see)** – Sometimes, you have to put on your detective hat to draw some insights about the person you're Facebook Creeping. For example, I once Facebook creeped a girl and she had a picture where she was

So, Where's My Girlfriend?

standing in the study room of her house. To the casual observer, the picture is simple: she's standing in the study with her overly mahogany furniture. To the trained observer however there is a wealth of information that needs to be unearthed for example: the bookshelf in the back. If you can see the books behind her, you may be able to derive some information as to what type of person she is. If the bookshelf is filled with Harlequin romance novels, then it might be a good idea to pick her up on your date riding a white unicorn. If her bookshelf is filled with books such as "The Joy of Sex", "The Kama Sutra" and "How to get laid for Dummies" then you might want to bring a condom for your date.

Bonus: if you find a novel in her bookshelf, read one page of that novel and during the dinner, bring up the novel and say *"you like that book? Me too! In fact, my favorite part is…*(insert that one page you read).

So the more diligent you are with your Facebook creeping, the more you information you'll have when you have a date with this person. The more you guys have things to talk about, the more you guys might like each other. In fact, she might like you so much that she might sleep with you on the first date…like what happened to me. To this day, I still think that she was 50/50 about me but my Facebook page was the one that tipped the scales in my favor. The lesson here is to fix your Facebook page.

At the same time that the Internet has helped people get laid, it also gives people time to get themselves out of rough patches during a relationship argument. You see, the Internet lets people buy time to think over what they want to say. A long time ago, the only two ways people could talk was either in person or over the phone (well, one can correspond through letters but do we look like we live in 18th century France?) If communication is made through the phone or in person, people literally have seconds to think of their answers during a conversation. That's fine if you're having a mundane conversation, such as:

Her: *How was your day?*
Him: *Good.*

So, Where's My Girlfriend?

Her: *Did you buy your lottery ticket?*
Him: *Yes.*
Her: *Did you feed your pet duck?*
Him: *No, he died.*

But during moments when conversations get hot and heavy, rapid fire answers may not be the best option. It would be difficult to answer the following questions in under two seconds:

"How can you say you love me when you look so lovingly into your secretary's eyes?"
"I used to be held lovingly one time by a man that used to love me...he doesn't anymore, does he?"
"Did the fact that you killed your duck have anything to do with your displeasure about my selection of wall paper in our new house?"

Clearly, these types of conversation require well-thought out answers. In the pre-Internet days, taking a bit too long to answer these questions may suggest guilt or incompetence. Lying in front of somebody's face is also possible but is really hard to do without looking guilty (i.e. shifty eyes or sweating like a pig). Now, given the emergence of the Internet, what humanity now has is…time.

Talking to somebody online affords people the freedom to do several things when working around tough conversations. First, since people can't see or hear one another through the computer, a person can actually get on the phone and call their friend for advice on how to answer tough questions, like the life line option in *"Who wants to be a Millionaire?"* If a guy needs a girl's perspective on something, then he can call his sister up. Secondly, if he can't think of a good answer by himself, then he can go on Google and cut and paste a philosophical quote to throw the girl off. I suggest something by Nietzsche or Barney Stinson.

Finally, if a guy really doesn't feel like answering any tough questions, he can just turn off his computer. This is the equivalent of hanging up on someone on the phone but this is even better. The guy can actually blame technology for screwing up – *"My Internet*

So, Where's My Girlfriend?

connection got cut off." This is a brilliant move as there's no way the girl can find out whether or not the guy is telling the truth - only the cable company knows his true intentions.

God bless the Internet.

So, Where's My Girlfriend?

Break Ups and all the Dirty Shit that comes with it.

So comes the part of a relationship no one really wants to talk about – breaking up. Unless you're one of the few lucky ones to never have to go through it, break ups are a painful part of any relationship and you might as well learn how to deal with it. The main reason you should understand and be comfortable with breaking up is simple: some people never get over a break up and it fucks them up for life. Not getting over a break up is like taking a piss in the town well: it ruins it for every person after you. If you don't get over a break up, you'll be carrying emotional baggage over to your next relationship thereby dooming it from the start.

So now I'll talk about some common reasons for breaking up:

Reason #1 - She's tired of his shit

When she first met him, she thought that it was cute that he spent every Wednesday playing poker with the boys. She also thought that it was cute how he wore his football jersey everywhere he went. Yup, he was a "real guy". Then, he realized that he really loved her and wanted to make her happy so he began to spend less time with the boys. Wednesday is now spent at the opera with her and he began to shop at Banana Republic instead of Footlocker. It clearly showed that he was willing to sacrifice a lot to make her happy. That's why he still has his hands up in the air in bewilderment when out of nowhere, she tells him that she's tired of his shit and she doesn't even know him anymore. He's changed.

In a relationship, guys are pretty much damned in whatever they do. The reason why a girl ever enters a relationship with a guy is because she wants to change the guy into her "ideal guy". Though girls will never tell him, they do it in subtle ways. She starts taking him to nice restaurants as opposed to the drive-thru he used to enjoy. She begins to shop for his clothes and introduces him to her gay hairstylist. These things are indicators that her project to mold him has begun. Ask any girl as to why she goes out with "bad boys" and she'll say that she hopes to turn the "bad boy" into a "good boy".

This thinking is shortsighted since girls never really ask themselves the real question: *What happens if they actually succeed?*

So, Where's My Girlfriend?

Girls are subconsciously masochists in the sense that they enter a relationship hoping to change their partners but in the back of their minds, they secretly hope that they never quite get there. There needs to be a constant tension within the relationship where the guy is uncompromising in some of his ways. Being uncompromising is the definition of being manly in society. When the guy begins to jump through hoops to make this girl happy, it's not that she's ungrateful of his efforts to satisfy her. It's just that she subconsciously begins to question his "manliness". To be uncompromising in some things is to show boundaries and limits. To let the girl walk all over him demonstrates the man's weakness. Being weak is not manly.

Looking back, it's not that she's tired of his shit, it's more like she's surprised at her success of changing him but is now tired of her creation. She will probably leave him for someone totally opposite...someone who's just like him before they met.

Reason #2 – He's tired of her shit

Comedian Chris Rock hit the nail right on the head when he talked about guys and cheating: **A man is only as faithful as his options.** It's a fact – guys are cold, callous and calculating. Usually, when a guy meets a girl, he knows right away whether she's marriage material, short-term fun or not worth his time. If she's marriage material, then he'll say and do anything he has to in order to win her over. If she's not worth his time, nothing she can say or do will convince the guy to desire her. That's also a big difference between guys and girls: with his persistence and efforts, it is possible for a guy to convince a girl to go out with him – this will never work vice versa for the simple reason that guys are assholes and they know that there will always be plenty more fish in the sea and that time is on their side. To recap: if a guy sees marriage material with a girl, he'll say and do anything to win her over. If she's not worth his time, he'll tune her out and move on. What about a girl who's only short-term fun? Here's the kicker: **if a guy only sees temporary fun with a girl, he'll say and do anything to win her over.** This means that a girl can never tell through a guy's actions what his true intentions are. This will lead the girl to think that this guy is seriously thinking long term with her leading her to trust him.

Going back to what Chris Rock said – a man is only as faithful as his options. So a guy meets a girl and sees her only as short-term fun. He wins her over and she's happy thinking that she's going to have a different last name in the future. All the while, she's unaware that she's only serving as a placeholder to any future girl that he thinks is better than her.

When you think about it, although it's morally reprehensible, the strategy behind this approach works: if the guy finds a better girl, he'll leave his current girlfriend. If no one else better comes along, he'll just marry her. She'll never know that she was the back-up plan. What a real asshole move.

Reason #3 – Sinking Ship: Everyone wants out.

Just like the Titanic, sometimes there are moments in relationships when both parties come to the realization that it's best to grab a life raft and jump off a sinking ship. As life is unpredictable, sometimes relationships which initially appear rock-solid suddenly become paper thin. I hate to use catchphrases but I really like this one: Shit happens in life:

- The guy might get a job offer halfway across the world and he has to move there but she's not willing to leave her family. Break up.
- Her parents don't approve of her boyfriend and she's not willing to go against the wishes of her family. Break up.
- He refuses to stop drinking, gambling and punching orphans. Break up.

So in this third reason, no one is being an asshole. Both parties just need to come to the realization that it's not going to work out and try to break up as amicable as possible. At this stage, it is crucial not to assign blame. They only need to know four words to make themselves feel better: **in life, shit happens.**

The Different Ways Guys and Girls Break up

Guys and girls break up in very different manners and for very different intentions. Girls my age (around 30) start to play for keeps and usually break up with their boyfriends when they don't see a long-term future with them. In other words, the guy is not marriage material. This is the main rationale for a girl to break up: short-term pain in order to avoid long-term pain. Usually, the girl breaks up with the guy thinking she's also doing the guy a favor and as a result, she's willing to play the bad guy and initiate the break up. To recap: a girl's break up style is simple and linear:

So, Where's My Girlfriend?

She sees a good reason to break up → Initiates break up → Starts fresh

Guys on the other hand do things very differently. To recall Chris Rock's observation: a guy is only as faithful as his options. So, we'll assume that a guy sees a better girl than his current girlfriend and therefore wants to break up. Sure, he can be a man and tell his current girlfriend why he's breaking up with her ("Honey, I found someone who actually likes reverse cowgirl.") but that's not the way guys operate. Remember earlier that guys are cold, callous and calculating? This is the calculating part – even before he even begins to hint at a breakup, the guy has already worked out the entire scenario in his head. More importantly, he's also worked out the implications and the aftermath of his break up in his head. **The guy needs to make sure that he doesn't look like the bad guy in the breakup because that will turn off future girls he meets.** Guys know that girls talk. If he's a total asshole in a break up, this will severely turn other girls off from him as girls are united in one thing: the feeling of shit in a breakup. As a result, if a guy's ugly breakup reputation precedes him, girls will not hesitate to send out warning signals to other girls about what happened with this guy before. As a result, the objective of a guy during a break up is to not look like the bad guy.

How does he do this?

Simple: provoke the girl.

Wait for a fight and use that reason to breakup.

How to Provoke a Girl to Break up with you

A good way to illustrate this point is to think of Franz Ferdinand, the assassinated archduke that started the First World War. The archduke's murder wasn't the main reason why the First World War started, rather a series of world events were already under way which readied the world for total war. His death simply got things in motion.

In the context of a break up – that stupid argument you just had about not tipping the waitress enough is the same as assassinating the archduke. Guess what: war was inevitable, the argument just set it off.

So the guy's been thinking break up for a while now and all he needs is a stupid argument to come his way. He finally gets it from you and when he does, he snowballs the argument from one isolated incidence to a general trait of your character.

So, Where's My Girlfriend?

Here's a very simple example:

Him: *I still think that you tipped the waitress too little* (isolated incident). *I mean, don't you care that these people are busting their ass to serve you? Are you that insensitive?* (suggesting that she possesses a negative character trait: being insensitive)

Her: *I admit that the tip was a bit small. I miscalculated.* (deflecting his suggested character flaw as situation specific thereby not reflective of her personality)

This is the critical juncture of the relationship – if he wants to continue dating her, he can agree with her and move past the topic. If he's committed to breaking up with her however he's not going to let go of the issue:

Him: *I don't know, this isn't the first time when you've been cheap. I don't know if I can see myself with someone who's so cheap…*

Her: *What are you saying? Are you saying that you don't see yourself with me? If you don't want to be with me, then what's the point of us going out? Maybe we shouldn't see each other anymore* (look! She just initiated the break up!)

After this crucial juncture, the rest is pretty much autopilot: argument leads to tears and tears lead to break up. The archduke is dead and the rest is history.

The Worst Part

We can see many obvious reasons as to why this approach to breaking up with a girl is such an asshole maneuver. The obvious reason is the dishonesty behind the break up: the guy doesn't want to pick a fight so he lets the girl do the dirty work. How this affects the girl is ten times worse – as she unknowingly falls into this trap, she will now always hold a sense of regret in her mind about the whole thing:

"If I didn't pick a fight with him about the tipping, maybe I would still be with him today. If only I tipped a bit more…if only…"

If only she knew that she never had a chance in the beginning.

So, Where's My Girlfriend?

The Aftermath

After the couple breaks up, friends will start wanting to know the details. More importantly, everyone wants to know: **who broke up with whom?**

The general rule is that the initiator is the villain of the break up because in North American society, nobody likes a quitter. The initiator of the break up is the one that pushed out women and children in order to get on the last life raft leaving the Titanic. Given the way the guy set up the break up, he made sure that it was a win/win situation for him. If someone asks *"Who broke up with whom?"* there are only two possible answers: either she broke up with me or we decided to call it quits.

The answer will never be: *I broke up with her* therefore he will never look like the bad guy. From what I recall from comic books, the best bad guys are usually the ones that don't look like bad guys.

Yeah, guys are assholes.

So, Where's My Girlfriend?

For more stuff:

www.sowheresmygirlfriend.com